THE

MAYO CLINIC PLAN

10 Essential Steps
to a Better Body
& Healthier Life

MAYO CLINIC

Medical Editor Donald Hensrud, M.D.

Publisher Sara Gilliland

Editor in Chief, Books & Newsletters Christopher Frye

Managing Editor Karen Wallevand

Contributing Editors Richard Dietman, Kevin Kaufman

Creative Director Daniel Brevick

Art Directors S. Jay Koski, Paul Krause

Proofreaders Miranda Attlesey, Donna Hanson

Indexer Steve Rath

TIME INC. HOME ENTERTAINMENT

Publisher Richard Fraiman

Executive Director, Marketing Services Carol Pittard

Director, Retail & Special Sales Tom Mifsud

Marketing Director, Branded Business Swati Rao

Director, New Product Development Peter Harper

Assistant Financial Director Steven Sandonato

Prepress Manager Emily Rabin

Product Manager Victoria Alfonso

Associate Book Production Manager Suzanne Janso

Associate Prepress Manager Anne-Michelle Gallero

Special thanks to: Bozena Bannett, Alexandra Bliss, Glenn Buonocore, Bernadette Corbie, Robert Marasco, Brooke McGuire, Jonathan Polsky, Chavaughn Raines, Ilene Schreider, Adriana Tierno

Published by Time Inc. Home Entertainment Books

Time Inc.
1271 Avenue of the Americas
New York, NY 10020

© 2006 Mayo Foundation for Medical Education and Research

ISBN: 1-932994-27-0
 978-1-932994-27-8

Library of Congress Control Number: 2005906439

First Edition

1 2 3 4 5 6 7 8 9 10

We welcome your comments and suggestions on *The Mayo Clinic Plan*. Please write to us at: TIHE Books, Attention: Book Editors, P. O. Box 11016, Des Moines, IA 50336-1016.

If you would like to order more copies of this book, please call (800) 327-6388 (Monday through Friday, 7 a.m. to 8 p.m., or Saturday, 7 a.m. to 6 p.m. Central time).

For bulk sales to employers, member groups and health-related companies, contact Mayo Clinic Health Management Resources, 200 First St. S.W., Rochester, MN 55905, or send an e-mail to SpecialSalesMayoBooks@Mayo.edu.

The Mayo Clinic Plan: 10 Essential Steps to a Better Body & Healthier Life is intended to supplement the advice of your personal physician, whom you should consult regarding individual medical conditions. This book does not endorse any company or product. MAYO, MAYO CLINIC, MAYO CLINIC HEALTH INFORMATION and the Mayo triple-shield logo are marks of Mayo Foundation for Medical Education and Research.

Photo credits: Stock photography from Artville, BananaStock, Brand X Pictures, Comstock, Corbis, Creatas, Digital Stock, Digital Vision, EyeWire, Food Shapes, Image Ideas, PhotoAlto, Photodisc, Rubberball and Stockbyte. The individuals pictured are models, and the photos are used for illustrative purposes only. There is no correlation between the individuals portrayed and the conditions or subjects being discussed. Photographs of Mayo specialists by Daniel Hubert, Richard Madsen, Siddiqi Ray and Randy Ziegler, Mayo Clinic.

Jacket design by Paul Krause.

Table of Contents

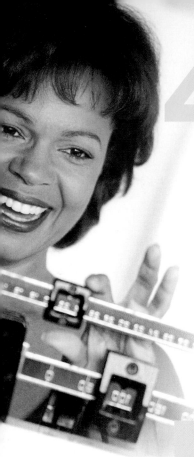
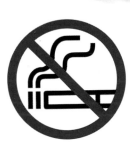

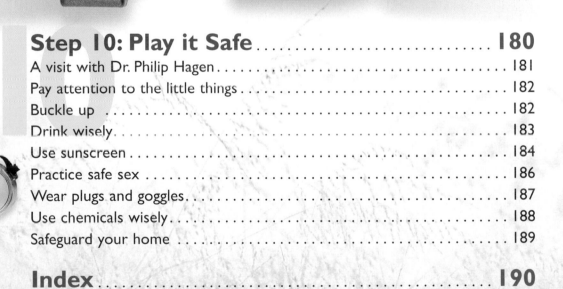

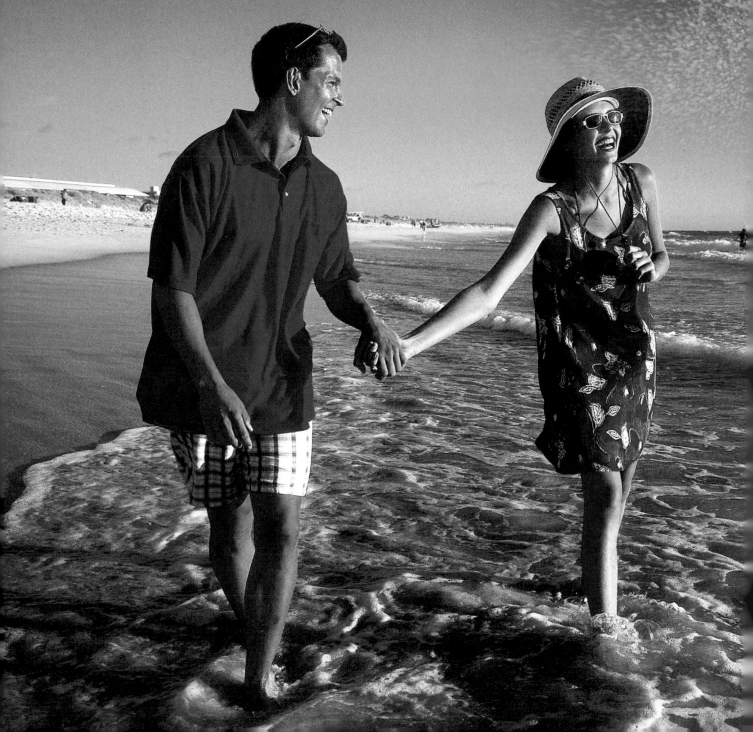

It's all about attitude

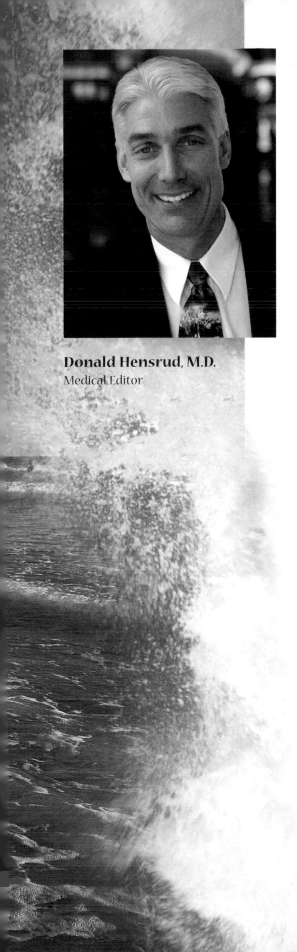

Donald Hensrud, M.D.
Medical Editor

Years ago, I asked a wise mentor of mine, "What's the most important factor to help live a long, healthy life?" I wanted to know if it was diet, not smoking or, perhaps, exercise. He replied, "None of those. ... It's attitude." I've seen his words validated many times during my years in clinical practice.

In this book are 10 key areas that you can focus on to improve your health and live longer. The pages that follow are filled with all sorts of tips and advice on the importance of developing healthy habits and how to make important lifestyle changes. Bear in mind that you don't need to make a lot of changes at once. Prioritize what's most important to you and go from there.

But as you may be well aware, knowing and doing are two different things. Just because you know that you should make some lifestyle changes to improve your health doesn't mean you'll actually make them. That's because behavior change is challenging for everyone. *This is where attitude comes in.* Having the right attitude can make all the difference in the world when it comes to putting knowledge into practice. A positive attitude opens the door, allowing you to challenge current beliefs, experiment with new routines and adopt new ways of thinking.

For example, I often see patients who want to lose weight. They come in to my office saying they have to "go on a diet." Their attitude is that losing weight is going to be drudgery — a negative and restrictive process. As a result, their diet will only be temporary and they'll soon return to their old habits. An alternative attitude is to focus on making enjoyable changes that will improve your health and help you feel better, instead of zeroing in only on the numbers on the scale. With this attitude, your chances of making sustainable and permanent lifestyle changes are much greater.

Sound too difficult? In general, people underestimate their ability to change. Most of you probably can think of changes that you've made in your lives that seemed very challenging at the time, but now they're a part of your daily routine. An example I like to use related to nutrition is changing from whole milk to 2 percent milk or skim. When people initially attempt this, a common reaction is that "low-fat milk tastes like water." However, if they can stick with it, they get used to low-fat, and their reaction changes to "whole milk tastes like cream." This illustrates that we shouldn't underestimate how much we can change and how we can adopt new healthy lifestyle habits if we approach change with the right frame of mind.

Read through this book with an open mind. Realize that adopting some of this advice may take some time, planning and effort, but it can be done. Starting out with the right attitude will not only help you adopt more healthy habits, but enjoy them. You can have fun and feel great while adding years to your life!

Step 1
Assess Your Health

A visit with Dr. Floyd Willis

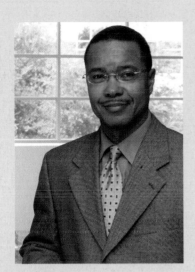

Floyd Willis, M.D.
Family Medicine

The majority of deaths in the United States each year are due in large part to preventable problems — conditions and situations that stem from our behavior, such as smoking, poor diet, minimal exercise, substance abuse and accidents.

To enjoy good health and reduce your risk of illness or death, you need to adopt good habits and reduce risky behavior. That said, what I'm seeing is that most people are interested in achieving good health, yet they often want to do it without changing their lifestyles or behaviors. It's nearly impossible to capture and sustain good health by taking a pill, taking a supplement or engaging in quick weight-loss or stamina-improving gimmicks. In today's society, people want positive results in an almost instant fashion. When it comes to health, I don't think that's possible.

I think the biggest obstacle to good health for most people is an unhealthy balance of exercise and diet. Exercise is powerful. By taking part in regular physical activity, you can lower your risks of illness from heart disease, stroke, diabetes, obesity, and a host of other problems. If you aren't very physically active, changing your lifestyle can be quite a challenge. But your efforts to increase exercise will provide a long-term payoff that's as valuable as any other effort to achieving good health.

Diet is part of a larger component to good health that I like to term *nourishment*. Nourishment has two very important parts. We should nourish "the body" with the right balance of food, as well as nourish "the soul" with relationships and activities that promote happiness and a sense of well-being. It's difficult to decide which of these two forms is most important, as they're often interconnected. If you don't include both to some degree, I think it's difficult to achieve excellent health.

Q: How reliable are height-and-weight tables in assessing overall health?

A: No single test or table can reliably assess overall health, but height-and-weight tables, such as the body mass index (BMI), can provide important information about how an individual's weight compares with others'. Though there's still controversy on this topic, many experts feel that underweight, overweight and obese people have greater risks of illness and possible death than do those who are "normal" weight. However, there are numerous disease risks unrelated to weight. Your health care provider can help determine which risks pose the greatest threat to your health.

Q: What are some key signs and symptoms that could indicate possible health problems?

A: Most governmental statistics suggest that heart disease, cancer, stroke and pneumonia are among the leading causes of death. There are several key signs and symptoms that may help us identify these illnesses. They include new or lingering pain — particularly chest pain — unexplained weight loss and fatigue, unexplained or lingering fever, and dizziness, numbness and tingling.

Often, you're able to explain why certain problems exist, such as back pain after lifting or recurring dizziness with known ear problems. New or lingering symptoms with no explanation should be evaluated by a health care professional.

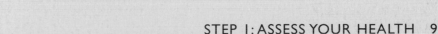

Gearing up

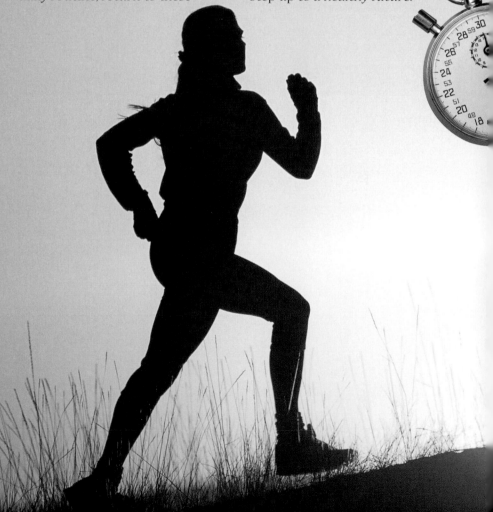

Contrary to what you may believe, genes don't always rule when it comes to your health. Health is influenced as much by lifestyle as it is by genes. Research confirms that while family history is important, your weight, activity level, stress level and health habits play a large role in determining your future.

What this means is that your future isn't predestined. When it comes to your health, you're in the driver's seat, and the sooner you identify and improve bad habits, the greater your chances of fully enjoying life.

On the following pages are four lifestyle assessments to help you evaluate your health habits and identify your health risks: Are you physically fit? Are you eating well? Are you bothered by stress? Are you getting enough sleep? Keep in mind that good health is more than good physical health. It also includes good mental health. Mind and body are intricately intertwined — the state of one greatly influences that of the other.

Use the results from these assessments to identify general areas or specific behaviors that you can work on to improve your health and put you on the path to better fitness.

For example, you may find that you're getting enough physical activity but your diet could use a nutritional boost. Or you may feel that stress and sleep are your problem areas. Because you're feeling stressed, you aren't getting enough sleep.

The steps you take now to improve your health will, over time, turn into sustainable, healthy behaviors that can improve your nutrition and level of physical activity, as well as enhance your overall well-being. Not only will you reduce your risk of disease and illness, you'll feel better and you'll look great!

As you make changes in your daily routine, return to these pages on a periodic basis to track how you're doing.

An important note: Don't view these assessments as a substitute for seeing your doctor. Regular exams are important because there are a number of health factors — your blood cholesterol and blood sugar levels and the health of your bones, to name a few — that you can't detect on your own. For a complete health assessment, you need the expertise of a health care professional.

Good luck as you begin your journey, and all the best as you step up to a healthy future.

Are you fit?

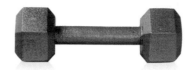

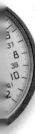

1 Do you have enough energy to enjoy the leisure activities you like to do?
- ① rarely, or never
- ② sometimes
- ③ always, or most of the time

2 Do you have enough stamina and strength to carry out the daily tasks of your life?
- ① rarely, or never
- ② sometimes
- ③ always, or most of the time

3 Can you walk a mile without feeling winded or fatigued?
- ① no
- ② sometimes
- ③ yes

4 Can you climb two flights of stairs without feeling winded or fatigued?
- ① no
- ② sometimes
- ③ yes

5 Can you do at least five push-ups before you need to stop for a rest?
- ① no
- ② sometimes
- ③ yes

6 Are you flexible enough to touch your toes?
- ① no
- ② sometimes
- ③ yes

7 Can you carry on a conversation while doing light to moderately intense activities, such as brisk walking?
- ① no
- ② sometimes
- ③ yes

8 About how many days a week do you spend doing at least 30 minutes of moderately vigorous activity, such as walking briskly or raking leaves?
- ① two days or less
- ② three to four days
- ③ five to seven days

9 About how many days a week do you spend doing at least 20 minutes of vigorous activity, such as jogging, participating in an aerobics dance class or playing singles tennis?
- ① none
- ② one to three
- ③ four or more

10 Approximately how many minutes do you walk during the day, including walking the dog, doing chores around the house, walking from your car to the office or store, doing errands at work, and going up and down stairs?
- ① less than 30 minutes
- ② 30 to 60 minutes
- ③ more than 60 minutes

How did you score?

To the left of the answer you chose is a point value — 1, 2 or 3 points. Add up the points from your answers to determine your total score.

A: If your total score was 26 to 30 points, congratulations! You're well on your way to overall fitness.

B: If your score was 20 to 25 points, you're on the right track, but your activity level could use a little boost. You'll find plenty of tips in this book.

C: If your score was 10 to 19 points, it's time to put getting in shape at the top of your to-do list. The pages that follow offer plenty of bottom-line advice to help get you moving more.

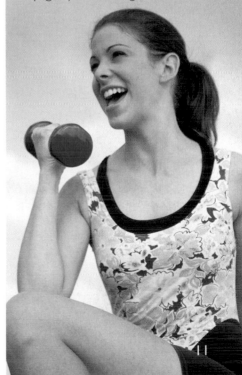

Are your weight and eating habits healthy?

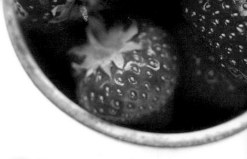

1 How do you score on the accompanying BMI chart?
- ① obese
- ② underweight or overweight
- ③ healthy

2 What's your waist measurement?
- ① considerably more than 40 inches (men) or 35 inches (women)
- ② 40 inches or slightly above (men) or 35 inches or slightly above (women)
- ③ less than 40 inches (men) or 35 inches (women)

3 Do you have a health condition, such as high blood pressure or diabetes, which would improve if you lost weight?
- ① yes
- ② possibly
- ③ no

4 Aside from holiday feasts, have you ever eaten a large amount of food rapidly and felt afterward that your eating was out of control?
- ① yes
- ② occasionally
- ③ no

5 Do you eat for emotional reasons, such as when you feel anxious, depressed, stressed, angry or excited?
- ① always, or quite often
- ② sometimes
- ③ never, or infrequently

6 How do your food portions compare with those of other individuals?
- ① much greater
- ② slightly greater
- ③ about the same

7 Do you sit down and eat three regularly scheduled meals?
- ① never, or infrequently
- ② sometimes
- ③ always, or most of the time

8 How long does it generally take you to eat a meal?
- ① five minutes or less
- ② between five and 20 minutes
- ③ 20 minutes or more

9 Do you snack a lot, or substitute snacks for meals?
- ① yes, or quite often
- ② occasionally
- ③ no, or infrequently

10 How often do you eat out at a restaurant?
- ① every day or almost every day
- ② two to four times a week
- ③ once a week or less

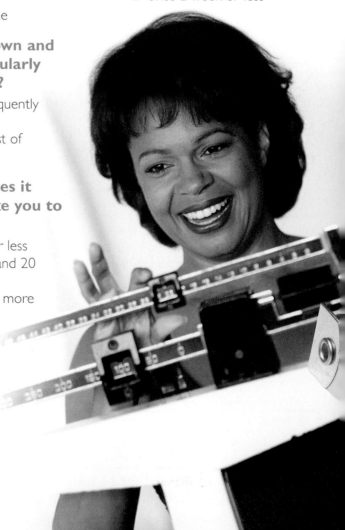

Body mass index (BMI)

You can determine your body mass index (BMI) by finding your height and weight on this chart. A BMI of 18.5 to 24.9 is considered the healthiest. People with a BMI under 18.5 are considered underweight. People with a BMI between 25 and 29.9 are considered overweight. People with a BMI of 30 or greater are considered obese.

BMI	Healthy		Overweight					Obese				
	19	24	25	26	27	28	29	30	35	40	45	50
Height					Weight in pounds							
4'10"	91	115	119	124	129	134	138	143	167	191	215	239
4'11"	94	119	124	128	133	138	143	148	173	198	222	247
5'0"	97	123	128	133	138	143	148	153	179	204	230	255
5'1"	100	127	132	137	143	148	153	158	185	211	238	264
5'2"	104	131	136	142	147	153	158	164	191	218	246	273
5'3"	107	135	141	146	152	158	163	169	197	225	254	282
5'4"	110	140	145	151	157	163	169	174	204	232	262	291
5'5"	114	144	150	156	162	168	174	180	210	240	270	300
5'6"	118	148	155	161	167	173	179	186	216	247	278	309
5'7"	121	153	159	166	172	178	185	191	223	255	287	319
5'8"	125	158	164	171	177	184	190	197	230	262	295	328
5'9"	128	162	169	176	182	189	196	203	236	270	304	338
5'10"	132	167	174	181	188	195	202	209	243	278	313	348
5'11"	136	172	179	186	193	200	208	215	250	286	322	358
6'0"	140	177	184	191	199	206	213	221	258	294	331	368
6'1"	144	182	189	197	204	212	219	227	265	302	340	378
6'2"	148	186	194	202	210	218	225	233	272	311	350	389
6'3"	152	192	200	208	216	224	232	240	279	319	359	399
6'4"	156	197	205	213	221	230	238	246	287	328	369	410

Note: Asians with a BMI of 23 or higher may have an increased risk of health problems.
Source: National Institutes of Health, 1998

FORMULA

You can calculate your exact BMI by using this formula:

$$\left(\frac{\text{Weight in pounds}}{(\text{Height in inches}) \times (\text{Height in inches})} \right) \times 703 = \text{BMI}$$

EXAMPLE

For example, if you weigh 165 pounds and you're 5 feet 10 inches tall, your BMI is 23.9.

$$\left(\frac{165 \text{ pounds}}{(70 \text{ inches}) \times (70 \text{ inches})} \right) \times 703 = 23.7$$

How did you score?

To the left of the answer you chose is a point value — 1, 2 or 3 points. Add up the points from your answers to determine your total score.

A: If your total score was 26 to 30 points, congratulations! Your weight and your eating habits appear to be healthy. Keep up the good work.

B: If your score was 20 to 25 points, you're on track but you may want to try to lose a few pounds, improve some of your eating habits, or both. You'll find plenty of tips in this book.

C: If your score was 10 points to 19 points, you need to make achieving a healthy weight and adopting better eating habits a priority. The pages that follow offer bottom-line advice to get you started on a healthy weight plan.

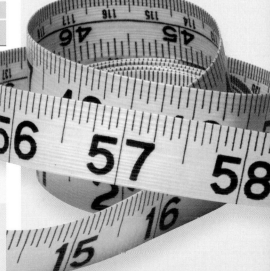

Are you eating well?

1 **How many servings of vegetables do you eat in a typical day?** (One serving equals 2 cups of leafy greens or $\frac{1}{2}$ cup baby carrots.)

① one or none
② two or three
③ four or more

2 **How many servings of fruit do you eat in a typical day?** (A serving is usually one small piece.)

① one or none
② two
③ three or more

3 **How often do you eat fish each week?**

① rarely, or never
② once
③ two or more times

4 **When you shop for bread, pasta and rice, how often do you buy whole-grain versions?**

① never
② sometimes
③ always

5 **Which of the following are you most likely to use in cooking?**

① butter or margarine
② corn oil
③ canola or olive oil

6 **How often during a typical week do you eat out and order hamburgers, cheese-rich pizzas or sandwiches made with meat and cheese?**

① four or more times
② two or three times
③ once a week or less

7 **How many times during a typical week do you eat a noon or evening meal that doesn't contain meat?**

① once or never
② two or three times
③ four or more times

8 **What kind of milk do you usually drink?**

① whole milk or none
② 1 percent or 2 percent
③ fat-free milk or soy milk

9 **What are you most likely to reach for when you're thirsty?**

① regular sweetened soda
② fruit juice
③ water or another calorie-free drink

10 **What's your usual snack?**

① chips, cookies or candy
② energy bars or other "healthy" sweets
③ nuts, fruit or raw vegetables

How did you score?

To the left of the answer you chose is a point value — 1, 2 or 3 points. Add up the points from your answers to determine your total score.

A: If your total score was 26 to 30 points, congratulations! You're making good choices and eating healthy.

B: If your score was 20 to 25 points, you're on the right track but your daily menu could use a tuneup. You'll find plenty of tips in this book.

C: If your score was 10 points to 19 points, you could use some fresh ideas about good food. The pages that follow offer plenty of bottom-line advice and even some recipes!

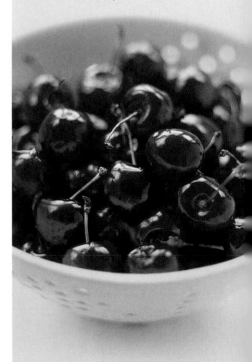

Are your other behaviors risky?

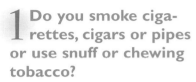

1 Do you smoke cigarettes, cigars or pipes or use snuff or chewing tobacco?

① yes
② very infrequently
③ no

2 Do you drink more than a moderate amount of alcohol? (A moderate amount is one drink a day for men age 65 and older and women and two drinks for men younger than 65.)

① yes, often
② sometimes
③ never, or infrequently

3 Do you wear a seat belt when driving or riding in a motor vehicle?

① rarely, or never
② sometimes
③ yes, always

4 Do you wear a helmet when riding a motorcycle or bicycle?

① rarely, or never
② sometimes
③ yes, always

5 How often do you use sunscreen with an SPF of 15 or higher outside in the sun?

① rarely, or never
② sometimes
③ always

6 Do you have working smoke detectors in your home?

① no
② most of the time
③ yes

7 Do you see a health care professional for regular checkups?

① no
② sometimes
③ yes

8 Do you often feel sleepy during the day and have trouble functioning because you're tired?

① often
② occasionally
③ never, or infrequently

9 How would you rate your ability to handle daily stress?

① poor
② fair
③ good

10 How often do you feel lonely, depressed or pessimistic about what's happening around you?

① often, or always
② occasionally
③ never, or infrequently

How did you score?

To the left of the answer you chose is a point value — 1, 2 or 3 points. Add up the points from your answers to determine your total score.

A: If your total score was 26 to 30 points, congratulations! You're making wise decisions regarding your health. Keep up the good work.

B: If your score was 20 to 25 points, you're on the right track, but there's room for improvement. Making just one behavior change could bring big rewards.

C: If your score was 10 to 19 points, your behaviors may be putting your health in jeopardy. Select one or two areas where you can make improvements and work on them. When you're ready, tackle another one to two items.

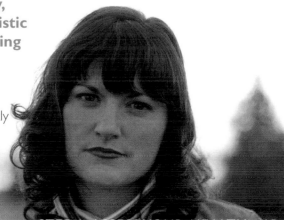

Step 2
Get Fit!

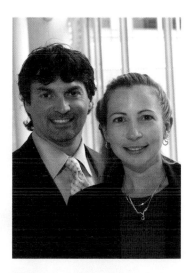

Husband and wife team
Diane Dahm, M.D.
and Jay Smith, M.D.
Sports Medicine

Being physically fit contributes to longevity, no question about it. In fact, improving your fitness is a more important factor in determining how long you'll live than whether you have moderately high blood pressure or are a little overweight. In addition, fitness improves quality of life, gives you more energy, helps you sleep better, combats depression and helps fight obesity.

If we were to recommend one activity that enhances fitness, it would be walking. Walk as much as possible, wherever and whenever you can. Things are too easy for us these days. We have moving sidewalks at airports, elevators, escalators, close-in parking. Unless you're disabled, walking is probably the easiest activity to do that requires only minimal planning and no equipment. And, of course, walking is natural.

We encourage people to engage in some form of physical activity at least 30 minutes every day. Fitness has such a positive effect in preventing or reducing the effects of a wide range of illnesses and conditions, such as diabetes, high blood pressure, high cholesterol — the list goes on.

We think exercising together as a family is a great way both to get and keep fit and to teach children the value of regular exercise. We get our kids involved in exercise — we swim together, bike together, go walking together. People often say they don't have time to exercise because they need to spend time with their families. The solution is to get the whole family involved in at least some aspects of your fitness program.

Q: Are there different types of exercise that are better for women than for men?

A: Not specifically. However, women face some health challenges to a greater degree than do men. Osteoporosis, for example, is far more prevalent in women than in men. Because of this, it's recommended that women incorporate weight bearing and balance exercises into their daily routines in order to maximize bone density and improve posture. Weight training activities also help maintain bone density and muscle mass, something older adults often lose as they age.

Q: Is it important to vary your exercise routine?

A: It's essential to periodically evaluate and vary your program. Your body may no longer be physically challenged by the same routine, and you may become bored. This can lead to burnout and lack of motivation to maintain your workout schedule. Keep your routine fresh by changing the kind of exercises you do, by varying the repetitions, by reordering the sequence in which you do the activities, or by changing the environment in which you workout. And try to avoid the trap of just doing more of whatever you're doing. It's easy to add more until you discover you've been overtraining and experience an injury.

The take-home message here is to look at changing something in your routine at least every four to five weeks.

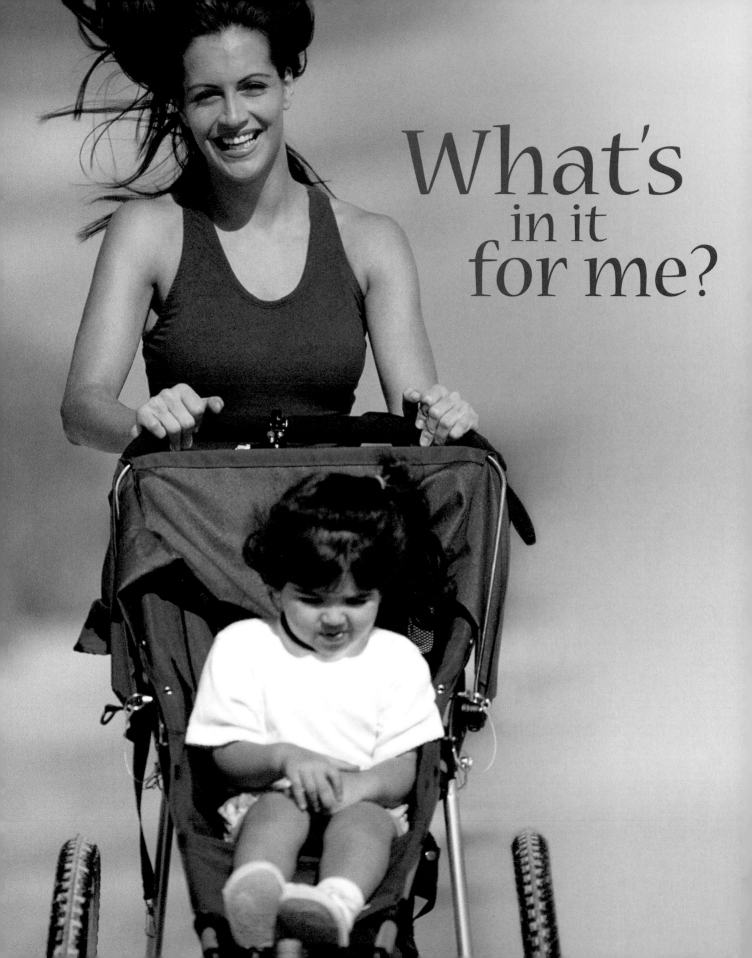

What's
in it
for me?

By introducing a moderate amount of physical activity into your daily schedule, you can significantly improve your overall health, well-being and quality of life. These benefits can be achieved by virtually everyone, regardless of age, sex, race or physical ability.

Whatever exercise you choose — and your activity of choice may vary from day to day — the key is to aim for 30 to 60 minutes of moderate-intensity physical activity on most days of the week. How you get it is up to you.

Don't like vigorous exercise? That's OK. Discouraged by trying to adhere to a strict exercise program? No problem. Physical activity takes many forms, a number of which you may already enjoy, such as walking, dancing, swimming, biking, skating, shoveling snow, raking leaves and washing your car. Almost anything that moves your muscles and gets your heart rate up qualifies.

The more you exercise, the more you may benefit. Even a modest increase in daily activity may help improve your health and quality of life. If you're already getting 30 minutes of physical activity a day, adding just one more mile to your evening walk or taking the stairs instead of the elevator at work may make your heart, muscles and lungs even healthier.

Almost anyone can exercise. Few people are too old, too young, too sick, or too busy to be physically active. Exercise is an equal-opportunity activity. People who are too tired to exercise often find they have increased energy after just a few regular sessions of physical activity.

Older adults can use strength training to reduce the risk of falling and breaking bones. People with chronic conditions can improve their stamina, mental outlook and ability to perform daily tasks with exercise. Truth be told, very few people have a valid excuse for not engaging in some form of exercise.

Adding more activity to your daily routine

Most of us have many opportunities for regular physical activity, but relatively few of us take advantage of them. Indeed, only about 22 percent of American adults engage in regular, sustained physical activity during their leisure time.

Although it's recommended that you adopt a regular exercise program, you can also make small lifestyle changes that add physical activity to your daily routine. By doing so you'll begin to experience some of the health benefits of increased activity. Consider these activities for giving each day a boost:

- Walk or bike on short errands instead of driving.

- Park at a distance from your destination and walk the rest of the way.

- Take the stairs instead of taking the elevator. If you work or live on an upper floor, take the elevator only partway up and walk the rest.

- Walk your dog. If you don't have one, offer to walk the dog of a neighbor or friend.

- Do your own yardwork. Mow your lawn, rake your leaves and shovel your walk.

Lifelong exercise

Were you on the college swim team? A 20-something triathlete? Great! But that's not necessarily going to ensure your good health later in life. Athletic participation as a young adult doesn't equal good health and longevity in later years. What does result in lifelong health and longevity? Maintaining physical activity and fitness throughout life.

- When it's practical, hold walking meetings at work instead of sitting at a table.

- While golfing, walk instead of riding in a cart.

Exercise fights disease and illness

When it comes to preventing and postponing the onset of disease and illness, one of the best tools is exercise. Regular physical activity reduces the risk of developing or dying of some of the leading causes of illness in the United States. By starting a regular program today, you'll help protect yourself against disease and illness, and you may find it easier to manage and control a disease or illness that you're already facing, such as those listed below.

Cardiovascular disease

Exercise helps reduce the buildup of deposits (plaques) in your arteries by increasing the concentration of high-density lipoprotein (HDL or "good") cholesterol in your blood. Accumulation of plaques in your arteries, caused by cholesterol and other products in your bloodstream, can interrupt blood flow and put you at increased risk of a heart attack or stroke. Walking as little as eight to 10 miles a week can increase your "good" cholesterol level, reducing your risk of cardiovascular disease.

Exercise also strengthens your heart so that it can pump your blood more efficiently and bring oxygen and nutrients to the rest of your body. It increases the flexibility of blood vessel walls and reverses hardening of the arteries.

High blood pressure

Fifty million Americans have high blood pressure (hypertension). Blood pressure is the force of blood pushing against the walls of your blood vessels. It's measured in millimeters of mercury (mm Hg) and is written as a pair of numbers. The first (top) number is the pressure exerted when the heart contracts (systole). That's your systolic pressure. The second (bottom) number is the pressure when the heart rests between beats (diastole). That's your diastolic pressure.

You have high blood pressure if either your systolic pressure is 140 mm Hg or higher or your diastolic pressure is 90 mm Hg or higher. People with high blood pressure have a significantly higher risk of heart and blood vessel (cardiovascular) disease, congestive heart failure, stroke and kidney disease.

Regular exercise reduces the risk of developing high blood pressure, even if you're already at increased risk of it. Most studies have found that not long after beginning an exercise program — three weeks to three months — blood pressure starts to decline.

Physical activity — both low and moderately intense exercise — also helps lower blood pressure in people who already have elevated blood pressure. Exercise has also been shown to reduce death in people who remain hypertensive.

Obesity

Obesity is a significant health problem in the United States. Many millions of adults ages 20 to 74 — 31 percent of the adult population — are obese. You're obese if you have a body mass index of 30 or greater.

In addition to the daily toll on your body and self-esteem, obesity carries with it serious health risks. People who are obese have an increased risk of type 2 diabetes (formerly called adult-onset or noninsulin dependent diabetes), cardiovascular disease, stroke, high blood pressure, abnormal blood fats, gallbladder disease, osteoarthritis, sleep apnea, asthma, certain types of cancer, menstrual irregularities and stress incontinence.

Coupled with a healthy diet, exercise can help obese people lose weight and achieve a healthy body composition, improving the problems associated with being seriously overweight.

Diabetes

Diabetes is a disease in which the body doesn't produce or properly use insulin. It's one of the leading causes of disability and death. According to the American Diabetes Association, 18.2 million people in the United States, or just over 6 percent of the population, have diabetes.

There are two forms of diabetes — type 1 and type 2. Type 1 diabetes results from the body's failure to produce insulin, a hormone that regulates the use of blood sugar by converting sugar, starches and other foods into energy.

Type 2 diabetes occurs when the body doesn't use insulin properly, allowing the concentration of sugar in the blood to increase.

A significant relationship exists between type 2 diabetes, obesity and a lack of physical activity. Approximately 90 percent to 95 percent of Americans with diabetes have type 2, and one in four older adults is at risk of developing it. Many are overweight and inactive.

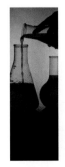

Researchers at the University of South Carolina in Columbia investigated the relationship between different levels of physical activity and the risk of getting a cold (upper respiratory tract infection). The study included 547 healthy adults between the ages of 20 and 70. Those who had a moderate to high level of physical activity experienced 20 percent to 30 percent fewer colds than did those whose daily activities were low.

Regular physical activity and a healthy diet reduce the risk of developing type 2 diabetes and can help control diabetes in those who already have it. This is because mild to moderate exercise helps insulin work better, lowering blood sugar levels.

Regular exercise prevents glucose from accumulating in the blood by helping muscles convert glucose in the bloodstream into energy. And by burning calories, exercise helps achieve and maintain a healthy weight, an important factor in the risk and management of type 2 diabetes.

Osteoporosis

Osteoporosis, a condition marked by decreased bone density and deterioration of bone, affects more than 25 million Americans. Bones affected by osteoporosis become weak, porous and fragile.

Because osteoporosis leads to fragile bones, it's a major contributor to bone fractures — a significant health risk for older adults.

Physical activity is likely the single most important influence on maintaining bone density. It plays several roles in preventing and treating osteoporosis. Perhaps most important is that exercise strengthens your bones.

Bones, like muscles, grow stronger when they're physically stressed through exercise. Weight-bearing exercises, such as walking and jogging, and strength training exercises, such as lifting weights or working with resistance bands, stimulate bone growth, increase bone density and protect against the decline of bone mass, making your bones healthier.

Fitness and longevity

In an expansive 20-year study of the lifestyles and exercise habits of 17,000 male Harvard University alumni, researchers established the importance of regular exercise. The study showed that moderately intense exercise — equivalent to jogging about three miles a day — not only promoted good health but added years to the lives of the participants. Here are some of the results.

- Men who exercised at the equivalent of a light sport activity had a higher life expectancy than did inactive (sedentary) men.

- Regular exercise countered the life-shortening effects of cigarette smoking and excess body weight.

- Those with high blood pressure who exercised regularly had half the death rate of those who didn't exercise.

- Men who walked nine or more miles each week showed a 21 percent lower death rate than did men who walked three miles or less each week.

- Regular exercise countered genetic tendencies toward early death. Individuals with one or both parents who died before age 65 reduced their death risk by 25 percent with a lifestyle of regular exercise.

- Men with the most active lifestyles — those who completed vigorous regular exercise — had the greatest life expectancies. This was due largely to fewer deaths from cardiovascular disease.

Exercise and immunity

Researchers have found a link between regular physical activity and improved immune function. With moderate exercise, immune cells circulate more quickly and are better at destroying viruses and bacteria.

Moderation is key. Some studies indicate intense physical activity — such as running a marathon — may lead to a suppressed immune system and increased susceptibility to illness, such as the common cold.

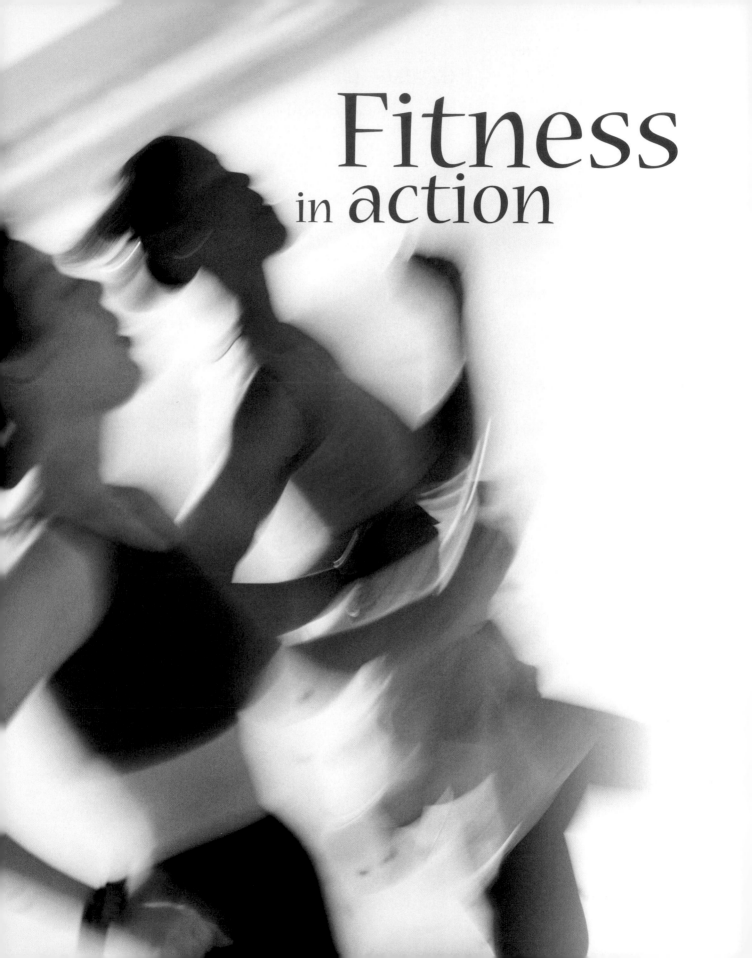

Fitness
in action

No matter what your age, aerobic exercise can strengthen your heart, blood vessels, lungs and muscles. And it can increase your stamina and endurance.

Aerobic basics

Aerobic exercise — low to moderately intense activities during which oxygen plays an important role in the release of energy in your muscles — includes some of the most popular, accessible and fun exercises you'll do, such as walking, jogging, dancing, biking and swimming. (See the Borg scale on page 24 for how to gauge exercise intensity.)

Walking

A brisk walk 30 to 60 minutes most days of the week can deliver many of the benefits of aerobic exercise. Even walking slowly can lower your risk of heart disease, although faster, farther and more frequent walking can deliver even greater health benefits.

When you gradually increase the amount of exercise you do, your body responds by improving its capacity for exercise and your fitness level improves. In just eight to 12 weeks, you may feel noticeable improvements.

Beginning a walking program

If you've been inactive and you have some health problems, see your doctor for a physical checkup and to discuss setting up a safe walking program.

Aerobic primer

- A beginning goal is to exercise at least three days a week and work up to at least five days a week.

- Before doing any aerobic activity, warm up for at least five minutes.

- Work toward a goal of exercising for 30 to 60 minutes daily, either continuously or divided into shorter sessions throughout the day.

- Spend at least five minutes cooling down at the end of your workout.

- Do some activity every day, even on busy days. If you can't fit in your regularly scheduled exercise, replace it with another activity.

- Take steps to increase your physical activity each day, even if it's not a scheduled exercise day. Jog in place while waiting for the bus or park a few blocks from your meeting and walk.

Aerobic workouts should include 3 stages:

- **Warm-up.** Before each session, spend five to 10 minutes preparing for exercise. This general warm-up should let you break a sweat but not be too strenuous. You can do the same activity that you do for exercise but at a slower pace. If you have a tight or previously injured muscle, also do some stretching of that muscle. Otherwise, save stretching until after your workout.

- **Conditioning.** Doing at least 30 minutes of aerobic exercise develops your aerobic capacity by increasing your heart rate, depth of breathing and muscle endurance. You'll also burn calories. How many calories you burn depends on how fast and how long you exercise and how much you weigh. The more you weigh, the more calories you'll burn.

- **Cool-down.** After each session, spend about five to 10 minutes cooling down. Stretch your calf muscles, upper thighs, hamstrings, lower back and chest. This after-workout stretch is important because it allows your heart rate and muscles to return to normal. It also helps develop and maintain muscle and joint flexibility.

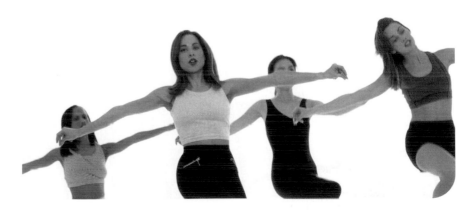

- **Start slowly.** If you try to do too much too fast, you'll likely wind up with pain and burnout. Instead, walk at a lower intensity for your first two to three weeks. Then gradually increase the intensity and length of your walks.

- **Establish a regular program.** If you simply decide to walk more, you'll likely find that your good intentions go by the wayside when your schedule gets busy. But if you make a commitment to a regular schedule of exercise, you're more likely to continue it. Plan, for instance, to walk Monday, Wednesday and Friday mornings from 6:30 to 7:00 a.m. Write it on your calendar and follow through.

- **Set goals.** Decide what you want to gain from your aerobic exercise program, then write it down. Make sure your goals are realistic and specific and include short-term as well as long-term goals. Instead of writing, "I'm going to start exercising," try writing, "I'm going to exercise three days a week by the end of this month, and five days a week by the end of this year."

- **Purchase the right equipment.** Good shoes are essential for your walking program. Although you don't need to spend a lot on shoes designed specifically for walking, do choose shoes that give your feet adequate protection and stability. And after about a year of regular wear — about 500 miles — you'll be ready for a new pair. To see if your shoes are breaking down, line them up side by side. Does either shoe tilt to the right or left? Have the soles started to separate from the uppers? If you answer yes to either of these questions, it's time to buy new shoes.

- **Dress appropriately.** Loosefitting, comfortable clothes are best for walking. Layers are recommended for most days because you can peel them off as your body temperature rises. Bright colors trimmed with reflective fabric or tape also are good choices. Wear sunscreen, sunglasses and a hat to protect your skin.

- **Don't neglect the stretch.** Make sure to stretch tight muscles, especially after walking.

- **Stay hydrated.** Drink plenty of water before and after your workout. Carry a water bottle with you if you walk for more than 20 minutes or if the weather is hot.

- **Take safety precautions.** Walk only in safe, well-lit areas, and consider walking with a partner. Spend time checking out your routes. Avoid a course above your ability level, such as one with steep terrain or uneven surfaces. Avoid trails or paths with cracked or uneven ground or narrow passages. Stay away from busy streets, especially at night, opting instead for sidewalks or walking paths.

- **Pay attention to your body's signals.** Although it's natural to feel some muscle soreness when you first start out or increase

Talk test

If you're unable to talk in short sentences while exercising, you're probably working too hard. Although you should be breathing hard or be slightly out of breath during your workout, you should also be able to speak in brief sentences. If you can't, slow down.

Borg ratings of perceived exertion scale

Perceived exertion refers to the total amount of effort, physical stress and fatigue that you experience during a physical activity. It's how hard you feel you're working. A rating of 6 on the Borg ratings of perceived exertion (RPE) scale is the equivalent of sitting in your chair, reading a book. A rating of 20 may be compared to jogging up a very steep hill. Ratings of 11 to 14 constitute moderately intense activity.

6	no exertion at all
7	extremely light
8	
9	very light
10	
11	light
12	
13	somewhat hard
14	
15	hard (heavy)
16	
17	very hard
18	
19	extremely hard
20	maximal exertion

Copyright 1998 Gunnar Borg

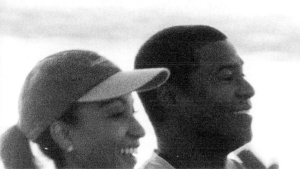

the intensity of your program, shortness of breath, a feeling that you can't catch your breath or joint soreness indicates that it's time to slow down. Walking should feel comfortable, not painful. If you have chest pain, chest pressure, heart irregularity, or severe shortness of breath during or right after exercise, seek emergency medical attention immediately.

- **Have fun.** If your walking program begins to feel like an obligation, take a day off. Then replace your scheduled walk with another activity that you enjoy, such as biking or dancing. You'll still get exercise and be able to return to your walking program refreshed.

A 12-week walking schedule

Try this sample program, in which you slowly progress in the frequency and duration of your walking workout.

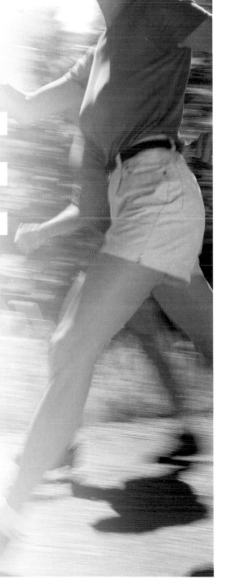

Week	Time (minutes)	Days a week	Total hours a week
1	20*	3	1
2	20	3	1
3-4	25	3	1.25
5-6**	30	3-4	1.5-2
7-8	35	4-5	2.5-3
9-10	40	4-5	3-3.5
11-12	40	5-6	3.5-4

*Older adults and people whose fitness is very limited may start out with just five to 10 minutes.
**If the days on which you can exercise are limited, you may choose to continue to walk three or four days a week but gradually extend each walk to 45 or 60 minutes. On the other hand, if you have relatively little time on most days, you may benefit from more frequent but shorter sessions.

This program can be adapted to many ability levels. A beginner might get a sufficient workout from a 10-minute walk around the neighborhood, and a more experienced walker can focus on increasing his or her speed, stride lengths or route, to make the workout more intense. Walking in a hilly area, for instance, may be a good choice for someone looking to boost endurance and build additional muscle tone in his or her legs. Note that walking with hand or ankle weights isn't recommended because adding these weights increases the stress and strain on your body.

Staying hydrated while exercising

Exercising or engaging in any physical activity that causes you to perspire increases your water requirement. Be sure to drink at least 1 cup of fluid before and after exercising and every 10 to 15 minutes during your workout. Water is all you need if you're exercising for an hour or less. If you're working out vigorously for more than an hour, have some fruit juice or a sports drink to replace carbohydrates and electrolytes. Drinking frequent, small amounts is better than drinking large amounts all at once.

Rarely, endurance athletes consume too much water and dilute their bodies' sodium — a vital electrolyte that helps the body use water to stay hydrated. This can lead to a potentially life-threatening

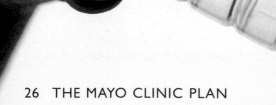

metabolic imbalance (hyponatremia). Signs and symptoms include bloating, nausea, incoherence, confusion, collapse and convulsions. Although this condition is rare, try to drink fluids that contain sodium and potassium, in addition to water — especially if you're running a marathon or performing in a triathlon or other prolonged event. These include sports drinks, tomato-based drinks and clear broth.

Energy and sports drinks

There seems to be an endless supply of energy and sports drinks from which to choose, all in a wide array of colors, from delicate blue to violent purple.

But are these drinks better for you than water? Not necessarily. Water is a great way to replace lost fluids, and it's inexpensive. Some energy and sports drinks may be useful in certain circumstances, and others may actually be harmful. Here's a brief breakdown from the American College of Sports Medicine.

- **Energy drinks.** These drinks usually contain large amounts of carbohydrates and caffeine.

Carbohydrates can boost energy, but too much caffeine, a stimulant, can have adverse side effects, especially if you're also on medications that contain other stimulants. Caffeine can make your heart beat faster, increase your blood pressure, interrupt sleep and cause nervousness and irritability. In addition, caffeine tends to act as a diuretic and can cause fluid loss rather than fluid replacement — not a good thing when you want to replace fluids.

- **Sports drinks.** These usually contain carbohydrates and electrolytes, which can enhance energy and replace minerals lost in sweat. Sports drinks can be useful if you've been exercising for longer than an hour and need to replace carbs and sodium. Some people find sports drinks easier to consume than just water.

- **Fitness water.** This is water enhanced with some vitamins, minerals, carbohydrates, flavoring and sometimes caffeine. The added value of any nutrients contained in these drinks is negligible in the amounts supplied. And the negative effects of caffeine should be considered before choosing a fitness water drink. However, if these drinks help you stay hydrated, then they can be useful.

Jogging

Jogging has become increasingly popular in recent years. Many people enjoy the challenge of training for local fun runs and road races, while others enjoy the role it can play in healthy weight management.

Start slowly. When you can comfortably walk two miles in 30 minutes (4 miles an hour), try to alternate walking and jogging — jog one minute, walk one minute — as shown in the chart at right.

Don't jog every day. In fact, unless you're a competitive runner, it's recommended that you don't jog more than four times a week — alternating days to minimize joint and muscle discomfort. Because jogging is a high-impact activity, spend one or two days each week cross-training with a low-impact activity. Participating in a lower impact exercise on these days will give your joints a rest while keeping your fitness level up.

During the program, it's important that you jog at a comfortable pace and walk briskly. Don't push yourself too hard — you'll be more likely to cause injury to yourself and to enjoy exercising less.

Cycling

Bicycling is a great way to add variety to your workout, and it may be better for you if walking or jogging causes problems for your joints. Many people enjoy cycling for its speed, its freedom and the opportunity to explore the countryside. Before you start, consider these tips:

- Always wear a helmet. They're available in a variety of colors and patterns.

- Warm up with easy riding. Save the hills and other challenging terrain for the middle of your workout.

- Try to keep your perceived exertion at the somewhat hard level.

Beginning a jogging training program

Advance one step in this starter program every two to seven days, as you feel able. If you're in step 1, jog for one minute, then walk for one minute. Repeat this until you've jogged and walked for a total of 24 minutes (12 repetitions). When you're comfortable with this portion of the program, move up to step 2. During this phase of the program, you'll jog for two minutes and walk for one minute. Repeat until you have jogged and walked for a total of 24 minutes (eight repetitions). Continue moving up in steps as you're able. By step 10, you'll be able to jog through an entire workout.

The whole program looks like this:

	Exercise time		Repetitions		Total time
	Jog	**Walk**	**Jog**	**Walk**	
Step 1	1 min.	1 min.	12	12	24 min.
Step 2	2 min.	1 min.	8	8	24 min.
Step 3	3 min.	1 min.	6	6	24 min.
Step 4	4 min.	1 min.	5	5	25 min.
Step 5	5 min.	1 min.	4	4	24 min.
Step 6	7 min.	1 min.	3	2	23 min.
Step 7	10 min.	1 min.	2	2	22 min.
Step 8	12 min.	1 min.	2	1	25 min.
Step 9	15 min.	1 min.	2	1	31 min.
Step 10	20 min.	—	1		20 min.
Step 11	25 min.	—	1	—	25 min.
Step 12	30 min.	—	1	—	30 min.

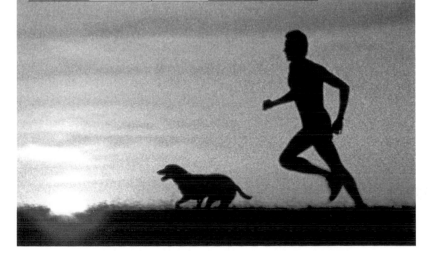

Fitness professionals' top-12 list

The American Council on Exercise asked 36,000 fitness professionals what they considered to be the most important exercise items. Their top-12 exercise essentials were:

1. Good shoes
2. Fun or appropriate music
3. Free weights
4. A positive attitude
5. Comfortable clothing
6. Lots of water
7. A supportive sports bra
8. Safe, well-made equipment, such as cardio machines and heart monitors
9. Weight training gloves
10. Enough time
11. A workout partner
12. Fresh, clean air and sunshine

Source: American Council on Exercise, 2003

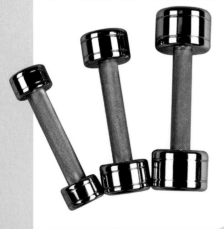

- When traveling, make stops for rest and fluids every 30 minutes.

To maintain variety and build fitness, the eight-week cycling program on page 29 includes different kinds of cycling — interval training, hills and different paces — over the course of each week.

At the end of the program, continue cycling by creating your own routine. Pull elements from this program and work toward a long trip with friends. Each day offers something different. By the end of the program, you can be comfortably cycling up to two hours and exploring biking trails that introduce new challenges and terrain.

Warming up and cooling down

Whatever your physical activity, no training program is complete without a proper warm-up before exercise and a cool-down afterward. Warming up and cooling down help reduce the risk of injuries and muscle damage.

A warm-up prepares the body for exercise. It gradually revs up your cardiovascular system, increases blood flow to your muscles and raises your body temperature.

Start your workout with a few minutes of low-intensity, whole-body exercise, such as walking, light jogging or pedaling on a stationary bike. It's often most convenient to choose a low-intensity version of your planned activity. For example, if you're biking, warm up by cycling at a slow pace.

After this light activity, take time to do any necessary stretches that are appropriate that target problematic areas.

Immediately after your workout, take time to cool down. This gradually brings down the temperature of your muscle tissue and may help reduce muscle injury, stiffness and soreness. Mild activity following exercise also prevents blood from pooling in your legs.

Cooling down is similar to warming up. After your workout, walk or continue your activity at a low intensity for five to 10 minutes. If you've been jogging, walk for about five minutes. If you've been playing basketball, you might cool down by shooting free throws. Follow this with stretching or flexibility exercises that are specific to your sport.

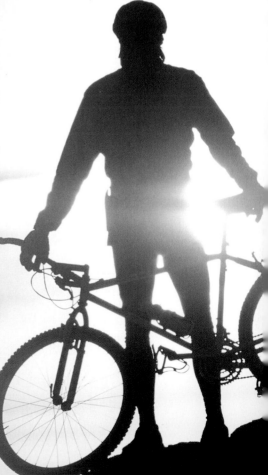

Cycling training program

Over an eight-week period, your cycling training program might look like this:

	Week 1	Week 2	Week 3	Week 4	Week 5	Week 6	Week 7	Week 8
Monday Ride at a comfortable pace.	30 min.	40 min.	50 min.	40 min.	50 min.	60 min.	70 min.	60 min.
Tuesday Cycle at a brisk pace.	2 × 10 min.*	2 × 15 min.	2 × 20 min.	3 × 10 min.	3 × 15 min.	3 × 20 min.	4 × 10 min.	4 × 15 min.
Wednesday Include hills to build strength and stamina.	15 min.	20 min.	25 min.	20 min.	2 × 15 min.	2 × 20 min.	2 × 25 min.	3 × 20 min.
Thursday Do interval training, pushing harder for brief periods.	3 × 3 min.	3 × 4 min.	3 × 5 min.	3 × 6 min.	4 × 3 min.	4 × 4 min.	4 × 5 min.	5 × 5 min.
Friday Go for distance, but take it easy to help build endurance.	60 min.	70 min.	80 min.	75 min.	90 min.	100 min.	110 min.	120 min.
Saturday	Cross-train. Try a different activity, such as walking, swimming or playing tennis.							
Sunday	Rest.							

*Note: Directions such as 2 × 10 min. mean do two 10-minute brisk intervals during the same exercise session.

Strength training basics

When it comes to overall fitness, investing in a set of weights or other strength training equipment may pay dividends just as great as those gained with a pair of walking shoes. The more fit your muscles are, the easier your daily tasks become, whether they include lifting children, mowing the lawn, shoveling snow or pushing a vacuum cleaner.

Strength training involves the use of free weights, your own body weight, resistance bands or a weight (resistance) machine to increase muscle strength and endurance. Adults of all ages can benefit from strength training. If you're inactive, you can lose up to 10 percent of your lean muscle mass each decade after age 30. If you do strength training, however, you can preserve and enhance your muscle mass.

Strength training can help you in a number of ways. Here are some examples:

- Strength training increases the strength of your muscles, tendons and ligaments and can decrease your risk of injury.
- Doing strength exercises increases the density of your bones, reducing your risk of osteoporosis. If you already have osteoporosis, strength training can lessen its impact.
- Strength training increases your lean muscle mass. This helps to raise your metabolic rate, making it easier to maintain a healthy body weight.
- People with chronic lower back pain often experience less pain after launching a program to strengthen their lumbar region and abdominal area. For many individuals, this significantly increases their ability to perform routine tasks.
- Regular strength training may improve your mental health.
- Because strength training contributes to better balance, coordination and agility, it can help prevent falls in older adults.
- People who commit to a regular strength training program have less insomnia.
- Strength training can improve your glucose tolerance and insulin sensitivity, lowering your risk of diabetes.
- Strength training has been shown to have a modest effect on decreasing the pressure in your blood vessels when your heart is relaxed (diastolic blood pressure).

Strength training safety

To begin a safe and effective strength training program, follow these guidelines:

- Always use proper form.
- Avoid lower body exercises with weight if you have had hip or knee surgery or replacement. Use the weight of your leg as resistance and discuss how to safely increase resistance with your doctor.
- When using free weights, aim for smooth, steady motions. Don't jerk the weights into position.
- Stop if you feel pain. Though mild muscle soreness is normal after doing resistance exercises, sharp pain, sore joints and pulled muscles are signs of injury. Joint swelling, is also a sign that you've overdone it.
- Don't lock your joints. Keep some bend in your knee and elbow joints while performing the exercises.

Getting started

You don't need to spend 90 minutes a day lifting weights to benefit from strength training. In fact, it's better that you not lift weights every day. Strength training sessions lasting 20 to 30 minutes and done just two to three times a week are sufficient for most people and can result in significant, noticeable improvements in just a few weeks.

Strength training is typically done in four ways — with free weights, body weight, machines, and resistance bands or tubing. A fifth method is plyometrics. You can choose one method or combine them for greater variety. Before trying any strength training exercises, it can be helpful to spend some time with a professional trainer who can help you design a resistance program and advise you on safety issues.

- **Free weights.** The term *free weights* refers to items such as

Did you know?

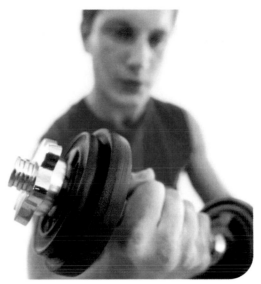

- Strength training, resistance training and weight training essentially mean the same thing.

- A previously unfit person can increase his or her strength 50 percent or more in six months with regular strength training.

- During strength training, the order in which you work muscles is important. The recommended sequence is large before small, multiple-joint before single-joint and higher before lower intensity exercises.

- Keeping a daily exercise log of your activity and progress is a great way to stay motivated.

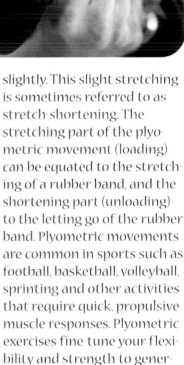

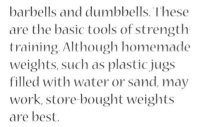

barbells and dumbbells. These are the basic tools of strength training. Although homemade weights, such as plastic jugs filled with water or sand, may work, store-bought weights are best.

When using weights, make all movements slowly and deliberately. If you experience pain in any of your joints when using weights, reduce the amount of weight or switch to a different exercise. When appropriate, such as when lifting heavy weights, use a spotter, someone who can take the weight from you if you lose control.

- **Resistance machines and home gyms.** These typically work different parts of your body with controlled weights and resistance. Some have stacked weights, others have bendable plastic pieces, and still others have hydraulic components. Each of these devices works by providing resistance to motion in one way or another. Most gyms will have a selection of resis-

tance machines to work muscles in each of your major muscle groups. Resistance machines must be adjusted to your height in order to ensure proper form during exercises. Overall, they're considered safe and easy to use.

- **Resistance bands or tubes.** These are elastic-like cords, tubes or flat bands that offer weight-like resistance when you pull on them. They come in different tensions to fit a range of abilities and are usually color-coded. Resistance bands are very portable and an inexpensive alternative to a home gym and can add variety to your workout. Remember that it's sometimes hard to determine the difference in resistance levels between bands just by using them, so make sure you understand the color-coding.

- **Plyometrics.** Plyometrics training is a specialized form of strength training that capitalizes on the ability of muscles to generate more force after they've been stretched

slightly. This slight stretching is sometimes referred to as stretch-shortening. The stretching part of the plyometric movement (loading) can be equated to the stretching of a rubber band, and the shortening part (unloading) to the letting go of the rubber band. Plyometric movements are common in sports such as football, basketball, volleyball, sprinting and other activities that require quick, propulsive muscle responses. Plyometric exercises fine-tune your flexibility and strength to generate large forces in short periods of time to do things such as jump, change direction and throw balls.

In order to successfully perform plyometrics, you must have adequate flexibility and strength. Consequently, plyometrics are considered advanced exercises that carry a relatively high risk of injury if not performed properly. The most common plyometric exercises include various hops and jumps that train the legs and lower body.

Free weights vs. machines — Which is better?

Ever since strength training machines came on the scene to compete with dumbbells and barbells, people have been debating the merits of free weights versus machines. Both methods of training have pros and cons, but muscle development occurs the same way whether you use free weights or machines. Your muscles don't know or care if the source of resistance is a barbell, a dumbbell or a plate-loaded machine.

Here are some of the advantages and disadvantages of free weights and machines:

- Free weights are much cheaper than weight machines.

- Free weights are more versatile. They can be used for just about every muscle in the body, while many machines have more limited functions. In this regard, free weights can be considered a better value.

- Using free weights generally requires more coordination and balance, compared with machines. Accordingly, for people with balance and coordination problems, the risk of injury may be higher with free weights than it is with machines, at least when they're first beginning to lift. Someone who's just starting a strength training program may be better off with a multigym machine, which is safer to use without supervision. However, if you're not at risk, you'll likely get more benefit from using free weights because they can more closely simulate real-life situations and they present a greater challenge to balance, stability and coordination.

- Free weights generally allow for more freedom of motion and involve several muscle groups at the same time. However, some machines can provide variable resistance, which means that your muscles work harder through a greater range of motion. In addition, some machines accommodate a larger range of motion for certain muscle groups.

- Weight machines enable you to isolate a muscle group, if this is part of your training goal.

- Machines can save you time — you can move quickly from one exercise to another.

- Machines may be easier to use if you're recovering from an injury, have balance or stability problems, or would be otherwise challenged by the need to control the free weight while lifting.

Free weights and machines will both do a good job of strengthening and toning your muscles. In the end, personal preference and comfort will likely dictate which type of resistance training you choose.

Major muscles first

Regardless of the method of strength training you choose, try to work all of your major muscle groups, including arms, shoulders, abdomen, chest, back and legs at least twice a week. Working each of these muscle groups regularly is important to avoid posture problems and strength imbalances.

You can perform a combination of exercises, but avoid exercising the same muscles two days in a row. Instead, plan to rest at least one full day between exercising each muscle group. This gives your muscles a chance to rest and recover from the workout.

Begin with a weight you can lift comfortably eight times and build up to doing 12 repetitions. Repetitions refers to the number of times you lift the weight or push against the resistance, if you're using a machine.

Once you have the appropriate weight, lift or push it into place as you count slowly to three. Hold the position for one second, then lower the weight as you slowly count to three.

Your movements should be unhurried and controlled. The weight you use should be heavy enough so that on the 12th repetition, you're just barely able to finish it with good form. For most people, a single set of 12 repeti-

Single vs. multiple sets

Are you confused about how many sets of strength training exercises you should be doing? Here's a simple answer. For most people, completing one set of eight to 12 repetitions, with the 12th repetition being difficult, is adequate. To progress, you simply increase the resistance. However, for someone who is looking to increase muscle mass and perhaps increase strength even more, adding a second set may be more effective.

Goal	Intensity	Volume
Strength	Moderate to high	Low — One set of 8-12 repetitions
Toning	Low to moderate	High — Multiple sets of 15-30 repetitions or work for 1-2 minutes at a time
Bulk	Moderate	Moderate to high — Multiple sets of 8-12 repetitions

tions with the proper weight is enough to build strength efficiently. You don't necessarily have to do multiple sets of each exercise to get the benefits.

If you're a beginner, you may discover that you're able to lift only 1 or 2 pounds or less. That's OK. Once your muscles, tendons and ligaments grow accustomed to strength exercises, you'll be surprised at how you progress. Avoid increasing weight beyond what you can lift with proper form.

You can develop a plan for working specific muscle groups on given days. For example, on Mon-

days and Thursdays you work your chest, shoulders, quadriceps and triceps — muscles that push. On Tuesdays and Fridays you can work your back, hamstrings and biceps — muscles that pull.

Strength training and women

Some women may worry about beginning a strength training program because they don't want to end up with large, bulky, body-builder muscles. But because of

Breathing while strength training

Breathing is something you do without a second thought. When you're strength training, however, you should spend some time thinking about your breathing.

Breathe normally through each exercise and don't hold your breath or huff and puff from too much strain. In addition, follow this simple guideline:

- Breathe out (exhale) as you lift, pull or push.

- Breathe in (inhale) as you relax.

For example, if you're doing biceps curls, breathe out as you lift the weight and breathe in as you lower it. It will get easier as you practice.

genetics, hormones and women's natural body types, this is unlikely.

Simply put, the average woman doesn't have near the testosterone of the average man and can't build as much large muscle mass. Most often, strength training helps women tone up muscles they already have. A women can experience a 20 percent to 40 percent increase in strength after a few months of strength training. As their strength grows, some women will experience a small increase in muscle mass. If this is a concern, a qualified trainer can help you avoid or minimize this effect.

Avoiding sore muscles

There's a name for that stiff pain you may feel a day or two after you push a little too hard during exercise. It's called delayed-onset muscle soreness, and it can be avoided.

The secret is gradual progression. As you increase the intensity, frequency and duration of your exercise, do so in slow, conservative steps.

For example, people who aren't used to exercising with weights should lift light weights just twice a week for the first month, and gradually build up to heavier weights and more days a week. Likewise, longtime exercisers who want to increase their workouts should begin slowly and work their way up.

If you do experience delayed-onset muscle soreness, light activity and stretching can help alleviate it.

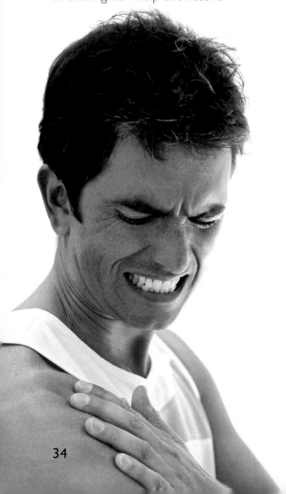

Core training basics

Core stability training is a type of strength training. It works the muscles at the center of your body. Added benefits of core stability training can be increased flexibility and balance.

The core of your body — the area around your trunk — is where your center of gravity is located. Your body's core links together your upper body and lower body. When you have good core stability, the 29 muscles in your abdomen, pelvis, lower back and hips work together.

In a very real sense, your core is your body's foundation. Core muscles stabilize the rest of your body and provide support to your spine, whether you're moving, standing or sitting.

Developing a strong, solid core gives you increased balance, controlled movement and a stable center of gravity that will help you improve performance. A strong core can significantly improve your athletic ability. It's the common link between your lower body, where forces are generated, and your upper body, where forces are applied by the upper limbs. For example, with a strong core you'll be better able to hit a golf ball, swing a bat, throw a softball, serve a tennis ball and shoot a basketball.

A strong core can also combat poor posture and low back pain, especially as you get older. For many, the prevention of low back pain may be the most compelling reason for exercising core muscles. As a result of sedentary lifestyles, it's estimated that 60 percent to 80 percent of Americans will experience low back pain at least once in life. Seventy percent to 90 percent of these people will develop significant back problems. Core exercises can help prevent and treat this problem.

Target your core muscles as part of your overall fitness program. While regular aerobic and strength training exercises also are important, most of these exercises focus on arm and leg strength without necessarily building a strong foundation of core stability. And exercises aimed at firming your abdomen, such as crunches, don't always reach the deep core muscles.

Examples of core training

Building core stability can be a lot of fun with exercises that add variety to your standard routine. Whichever core exercises you choose, aim to do them three times a week, or every other day.

Essentially any exercise that uses the trunk of your body without support is a core exercise. For example, a push-up stresses your core more than does a bench press, during which the bench is supporting your trunk. As a result, nearly any exercise can be modified to increase your core activity and strengthen core muscles.

It's a good idea to get some personal instruction as you begin a core training program because pinpointing your core muscles takes some practice. Taking a class with a certified fitness instructor can help you make sure you're using the correct muscles. In addition, a number of videotapes and DVDs are available to help you learn the various exercises, such as these:

Fitness ball workouts

Fitness balls, which look like large, sturdy beach balls, can be used to work the deep core muscles of your abdomen and back. If you're stocking a home gym, fitness balls are versatile investments. They're also called stability balls, physioballs or Swiss balls — because they were first used in Switzerland many years ago to help rehabilitate people with stroke-related disabilities. These balls not only work the trunk in almost every exercise they're designed for, but also help with balance and flexibility exercises.

When strengthening your core with a fitness ball, you'll want to create a balance between your abdominal muscles and your back muscles by doing exercises that work each equally. This is because if either your abdomen or your back is significantly stronger than the other, your body will be pulled in that direction. This can lead to pain and poor posture. Practicing the proper exercises with a stability ball can help you develop and strengthen all core muscles, alleviating this problem.

Pilates

With its recent surge in popularity, you might think that Pilates is a hot new exercise fad. In truth, Pilates is a low-impact fitness technique developed back in the 1920s by Joseph Pilates. Designed to strengthen the body's core muscles by developing pelvic stability and abdominal control, Pilates exercises also help improve flexibility, joint mobility and strength. They can help you develop long, strong muscles, maintain a strong back and improve your posture.

Many Pilates exercises are done with special machines. The earliest Pilates machine, called the Reformer, was a wooden contraption outfitted with cables, pulleys, springs and sliding boards. Using their own body weight as resistance, exercisers used the Reformer to perform a series of range-of-motion exercises that worked the abdominals, back, upper legs and buttocks.

Although machines are still used, many Pilates programs offer floor-work classes as well, designed to stabilize and strengthen the core back and abdominal muscles. Instead of emphasizing quantity, Pilates focuses on quality, meaning that exercisers do very few, but extremely precise, repetitions.

Floor exercises

Some common exercises that you already may be doing, such as squats, step-ups and push-ups, help strengthen your core muscles.

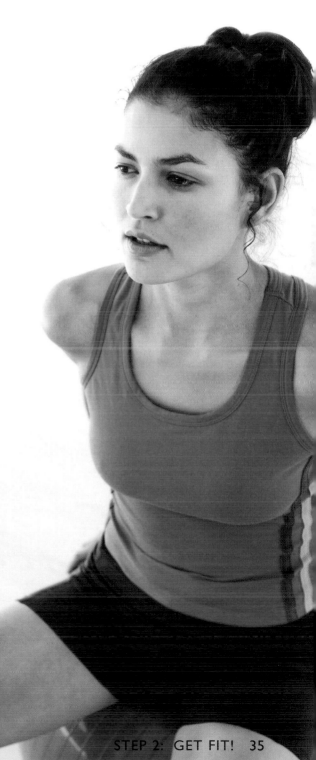

Flexibility basics

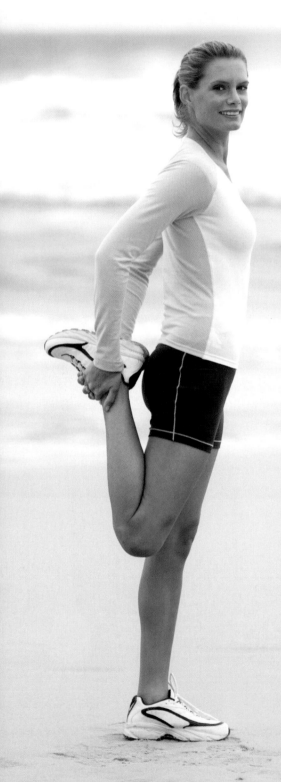

When you hear the terms *flexible* and *agile*, you may think of Olympic gymnasts or world-class ballerinas. But the truth is that everyone is flexible to some degree, and almost anyone can acquire greater flexibility. Flexibility is the ability to move your joints through their full range of motion.

Try to incorporate warm-up activities and cool-down stretches into your aerobic or strength training exercises. This is especially important for problem areas, like stiff or previously injured muscles. It's generally best to stretch problem areas after you exercise.

In addition to stretching after exercise, you may want to adopt a stretching program. A three-day-a-week program focuses on major muscle groups, including calf, thigh, hip, lower back, neck and shoulder. You may also want to stretch any muscles and joints that you routinely use at work or play. For example, if you frequently play tennis or golf, working in a few extra shoulder stretches loosens the muscles around your shoulder joint, making it feel less tight and more ready for action.

Before stretching, take a few minutes to warm your muscles. Stretching muscles when they're cold increases your risk of injury. Warm up by walking while gently swinging your arms, or do a favorite low-intensity exercise for at least five minutes.

Stretching techniques are fairly simple and easy to learn. Here are some general guidelines:

- Hold your stretches for at least 30 seconds and up to a minute for a really tight muscle or problem area. That can seem like a long time, so use a watch. For most of your muscle groups, if you hold the stretches for at least 30 seconds, you'll need to do each stretch only once or twice.

- Begin with an easy stretch of about 15 seconds. Stretch until you feel a mild tension, then relax as you hold the stretch longer. The tension should be comfortable, not painful.

- Once you've completed the easy stretch, stretch just a fraction of an inch farther until you again feel mild tension. Hold it for 15 seconds. Again, you should feel tension, but not pain.

- Relax and breathe freely while you're stretching. Try not to hold your breath. Exhale as you bend forward and then breathe slowly as you hold the stretch.

- Avoid bouncing. This can cause small tears in muscle, which leave scar tissue as the muscle heals. The scar tightens the muscle further, making you even less flexible.

- Focus on pain-free stretching. If you feel pain you've gone too far. Back off to where you don't feel any pain. That's where you'll want to hold the stretch.

- Avoid locking your joints.

Balance basics

Balance is your ability to control your center of gravity over your base of support. When standing, your base of support is the feet — or foot — you have on the ground. Balance is related to your strength, inner ear balance center (vestibular system), vision, and sensory input from your feet, as well as muscles and tendons.

Balance exercises can help you maintain your balance — and confidence — at any age. They can help you reduce falls, improve your coordination and give you more confidence in your stability.

When combined with strength training, balance exercises can help you build muscles around your joints, making them more stable and your balance more sure. People who do balance exercises have greater mobility as they age.

Examples of balance training

Almost any activity that keeps you on your feet and moving is helpful in maintaining good balance. Basic exercises that get your legs and arms moving at the same time can help you maintain your balance in addition to stimulating muscle and nerve communication that increases your coordination.

Muscles and tendons have sensory receptors — called proprioceptors — that play a key role in balance. Proprioceptors sense changes in muscle and tendon tension and pressure and relay that information to the central nervous system.

Proprioceptive training is a specialized form of balance training that deliberately challenges your balance in increments, similar to the way adding more weight challenges muscles in strength training. Proprioceptive training helps increase your ability to balance and to regain your balance. For example, ankle proprioception helps you avoid sprains when hiking on uneven surfaces.

Anytime, anywhere

Although it's important to incorporate balance exercises into your regular exercise program, you can also incorporate them into your daily routine. Consider these balance exercises to practice throughout your day:

- Balance on one foot and then the other while waiting for the bus, doing the dishes, brushing your teeth or standing in line at the grocery store.

- Stand up and sit down without using your hands. The nice thing about this exercise is that you'll have a chair right there to catch you if you lose your balance.

- Do the balance walk. Place your heel just in front of the toes of your opposite foot with each step. Make sure your heel and toes touch or almost touch.

Two-for-ones

One of the best ways to build balance is by walking. So while you're out getting your aerobic exercise with a brisk walk, you're also improving your balance. Walking keeps your leg muscles strong and reinforces your basic balance.

You can also save time by incorporating balance exercises with your strength training. Just add the following variations to strength exercises, such as standing on one leg, using a weight in only one hand, or standing on a pillow or foam pad while performing an exercise.

For each of these variations, make sure someone is nearby to help you in case you lose your balance, or put yourself in position to hold on to a rail or stable surface if needed.

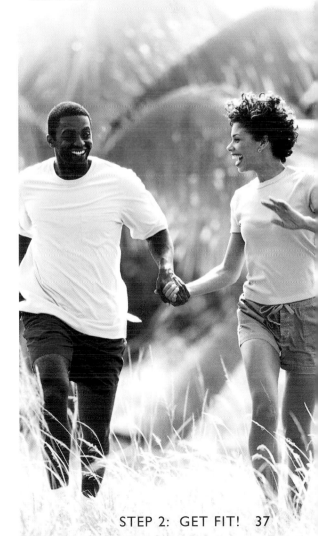

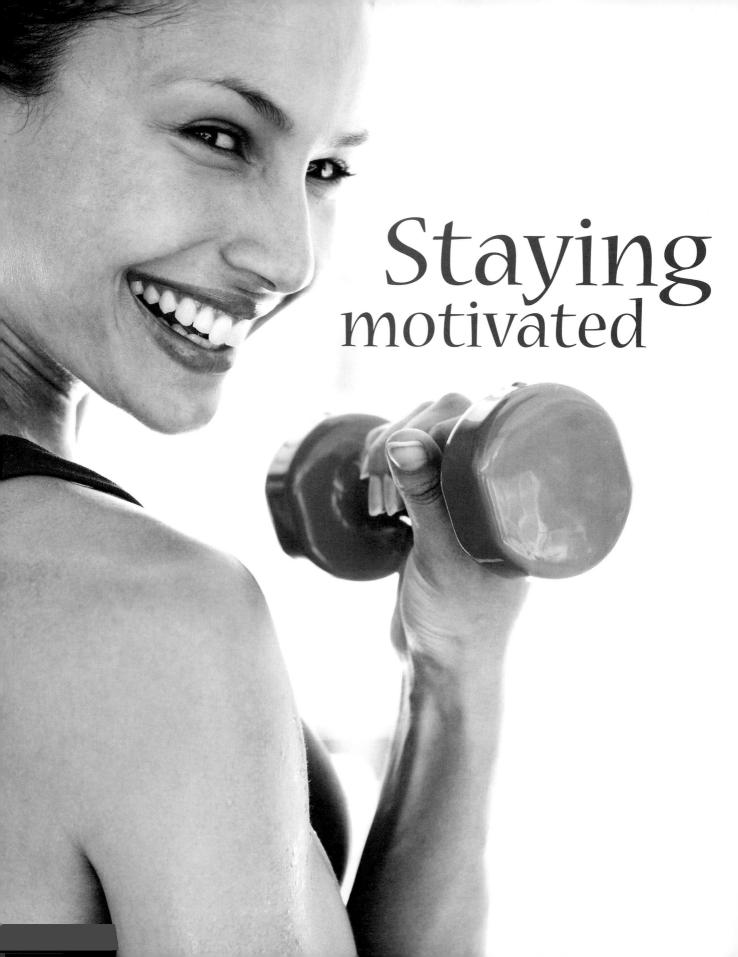

Staying
motivated

Even if you've never stuck to an exercise program before, you can do it. The following tips will help you stay motivated for the long haul.

- **Start slowly.** The most common mistake is starting a fitness program at too high an intensity and progressing too quickly. If your body isn't accustomed to vigorous exercise, your joints, ligaments and muscles are more vulnerable to injury. It's often not until the next day that you discover you've overdone it, and the resulting pain and stiffness can be very discouraging.

  It's better to progress slowly than to push too hard and be forced to abandon your program because of pain or injury. You can increase your activity in a deliberate way, but you don't have to be regimented about it. Taking small steps to increase your activity brings fitness benefits. For example, if you start out walking 10 minutes three times a week and extend each walk by just three minutes a week, in three months you will be walking more than 45 minutes during each outing.

- **Make a commitment.** It takes about three months to develop a healthy habit. If you can keep at your fitness program faithfully for that long, you're more likely to stay with it for the long term.

- **Accept some ambivalence.** Everyone who embarks on a major lifestyle change feels ambivalent about it at some

Talk yourself up

Whenever you think about something, you are, in a sense, talking to yourself. Psychologists refer to this as self-talk. Becoming conscious of what you're saying to yourself and making it more positive can help you break bad habits, boost your self-confidence and encourage you to stick with your exercise program.

Positive self-talk can increase your energy and motivation and help you remain physically active, while negative self-talk is critical and anxiety producing and can derail your efforts to get fit. One proven technique for overcoming self-defeating self-talk is to replace negative thoughts with positive ones. Here are some examples:

Negative self-talk	Positive self-talk
• I'm so tired.	• I'm going to feel more energized.
• I should be better at this by now.	• I've made some real improvements and am where I need to be.
• Skipping this one walk won't matter.	• Every little bit makes a big difference.
• I'll never stick with this exercise program.	• Just take one day at a time and have fun.
• I'll never recover from this injury.	• Healing takes time. I'll just continue to do something every day.

You can also use self-talk to break old habits and create new automatic responses. If you golf, for example, you can improve your form by saying things such as "Arm straight" or "Head down." Over time, as you reprogram your self-talk, the positive thoughts will be more automatic.

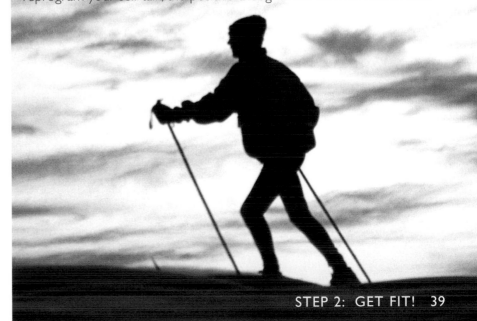

Excuse busters

Do you have the perfect excuse not to exercise? Here's the truth about some common "I can't because …" excuses. Yes, you can!

Excuse: I don't have time to exercise.

This is the all-time favorite excuse, but with some planning, you can make time for fitness. Most people have more free time than they realize. For example, the average American watches more than four hours of television each day. Add to that the time you spend reading the newspaper and surfing the Web. Remember, exercise is more important for your health than most anything else in your day.

Excuse: I'm too old to exercise.

You're never too old to be physically active, and it's never too late to start. Even moderate physical activity, such as walking or raking leaves, can help prevent or delay age-associated conditions such as heart disease, diabetes, high blood pressure and bone loss. Strength training can help prevent falls and maintain bone density.

Excuse: I'm too tired to exercise.

Maybe that's because you're not exercising. Regular physical activity gives you more energy. Fatigue is often more mental than physical and may be related to stress. A brisk walk, tennis game or bike ride can relieve tension and be energizing.

Excuse: I can't exercise because I have a chronic health condition.

This excuse is only valid if your doctor has told you not to exercise. Physical activity can help you better manage symptoms of many chronic conditions. For example, if you have arthritis, proper exercise can help you maintain joint mobility. If you have diabetes, exercise helps lower your blood sugar levels.

Excuse: I can't exercise because I'm too out of shape.

This doesn't cut it. You may not be able to run a mile, but you can walk a block or two. Start small and gradually increase your activity level. Pretty soon you won't be out of shape.

Excuse: I'm not overweight, so I don't need to exercise.

Being thin doesn't necessarily mean you're fit. Although a healthy weight is important, it's also important that your body get regular exercise. Inactivity, even when you're not overweight or obese, is a risk factor for chronic conditions such as diabetes, high blood pressure, stroke and cardiovascular disease.

point. Even regular, committed exercisers occasionally have days when they'd rather stay in bed than get up and work out. Ambivalent thoughts don't have to be more than a passing detour.

- **Broaden your definition of physical activity.** Physical activity doesn't just mean working out for 40 minutes or running several miles. Everyday activities such as walking the dog, biking to the store or taking the stairs at work promote health, too. Doing something daily is what counts.

- **Choose activities you enjoy.** Boredom is a major reason people stop exercising. If you have to drag yourself to a gym or you find walking on a treadmill mind-numbingly dull, then you're going to seize on any possible excuse to avoid these activities. Instead of beating yourself up about your lack of motivation, find activities you like doing. Consider joining a health club, at least on a temporary basis, so that you can try out many different activities.

- **Choose activities that fit your lifestyle.** Do you like to exercise alone or with a group? If you prefer solitude, consider walking, jogging or biking. If group activities appeal to you, consider enrolling in a yoga or dance class or joining a league or team for golf, basketball or softball. If you normally watch the evening news, walk on a treadmill, do balance exercises or lift free weights in front of the television.

- **Learn discipline.** To make a permanent change, you have to consciously build your discipline "muscle." Practice with small steps. For example, tell yourself you'll use the stairs at work today. Then do it, even if you change your mind and don't feel like it. Eventually, your discipline will pay off in the form of new habits.

- **Plan for exercise.** Reserve a time slot each day for physical activity, and protect that time. If you wait to find the time, you probably won't do it. Schedule an exercise appointment just as you would a haircut or an important meeting.

- **Avoid all-or-nothing thinking.** If you don't have time to run your usual four miles or to spend 30 minutes lifting weights, do what you can — a brisk one-mile walk, some wall push ups and other at home strength exercises. On days when time is tight or your motivation is waning, do less, but do something.

- **Remember how good it feels.** When you find yourself dragging your feet, call to mind the thought of how great you feel after an exercise session. Use images of successful experiences that remind you of how good physical activity makes you feel.

- **Savor your transformation.** Many people are amazed to find that the exercise they've been dreading for all these years is actually quite pleasant. Once you've been active for a while, you may find that you're stronger and more fit, which translates to a host of benefits.

- **Be patient and flexible.** When you can't perform your usual exercise routine because of illness, injury, travel or demands on your time, don't let guilt paralyze you further. Instead, adapt your exercise program to accommodate your schedule. A brief period of decreased activity isn't a disaster. Just get going again as soon as possible and return to your previous fitness routine.

- **Keep an exercise log.** Record what you do each day. Keep the log in a handy place. It will help you track your progress.

- **Affirm your efforts with words and images.** What you think affects your fitness plan almost as much as what you do. Negative thoughts can keep you from exercising and positive thoughts or affirmations can keep you going.

- **Use guided imagery to help boost your motivation.** In a state of concentrated awareness, imagine yourself getting ready to exercise. Picture obstacles that might keep you from working out, and then picture yourself overcoming each of them. Imagine yourself exercising and enjoying it, feeling energized and reaching your goals.

- **Support your plan with other healthy behaviors.** In addition to exercising, get adequate sleep. Sleep reduces fatigue and helps you recover from injury and illness. Drink plenty of fluids and eat a variety of healthy foods. Reduce stress and if you smoke, stop.

Injury

Each year, an estimated 7 million Americans receive medical attention for sports- or recreation-related injuries. Although two-thirds of these injuries happen in young people, adults aren't exempt — one-quarter of the injuries occur among 24- to 44-year-olds, and sports-related injuries among people age 65 and older have increased significantly in the last 15 years.

Most exercise-related injuries affect the upper and lower extremities — ankles, feet, lower legs, hands, wrists and shoulders. Low back injuries also are common.

Strains and sprains are the most common exercise-related injuries, followed by fractures. These injuries typically occur as a result of a fall, overexertion, hitting something or being hit.

One of the major risk factors for exercise and sports injuries is level of fitness. In general, the less fit you are, the greater your chance of getting hurt. Age is another factor. Older adults' muscles and tendons are more susceptible to injury. This is why it's so important to begin any new physical activity or exercise program at low duration and intensity and build up gradually.

Plateaus

You've been working out for a few months, and you're not seeing the same kind of results as you did in the beginning. What's going on? You may have hit a plateau in your fitness program. This sense of running into a wall is familiar to many exercisers. Unless you update your program regularly, you'll likely come to a plateau at some point along your journey.

Plateaus can happen for several reasons. One is physiologic. After several weeks of working out at the same intensity and duration or lifting the same amount of weight with the same number of reps, your body adapts to that level of activity. You won't see continued improvements unless you alter your routine to reflect the changes in your body.

Sometimes you reach a plateau when you're bored or losing interest in an activity. Or you may hit a plateau if you're overtraining — working out too hard or too frequently.

A plateau doesn't have to be a pitfall. If you find yourself stalling out, first figure out the cause of the plateau and then determine an appropriate solution. Are you overtraining? Have you reach a physiologic plateau? If the problem appears to be physiologic, you may need to increase the frequency, duration or intensity of your activity. But doing more may not be an option. For example, you may not have the extra time to commit to exercising. In this case, try the following strategies:

Preventing an injury

Most injuries that occur during physical activity stem from the "terrible toos" — too much, too hard, too fast, too soon, too long. A novice runner who struggles to complete five miles the first time out likely will hurt afterward. The couch potato who comes to life for the annual company softball game is an excellent candidate for a sprain, strain or other type of injury.

To minimize your chances of getting hurt, follow these guidelines:

- Follow the 10 percent rule. Limit the increases in duration and intensity of your training to 10 percent. For example, if you swim laps for 30 minutes this week, increase to 33 minutes next week, and so on.

- Warm up.

- Start out slowly and exercise at the appropriate intensity.

- Get adequate sleep.

- Keep your muscles conditioned through regular activity. Avoid being a weekend warrior.

- If your muscles are sore, ease up on your exercise routine.

- A previous injury increases your risk of a subsequent one, so if you've been injured before, talk with your doctor about appropriate physical activities.

- Use proper form and technique.
- Wear proper shoes and protective equipment.
- Take appropriate precautions for the weather conditions.
- Drink plenty of water.
- Use pain relievers with caution because they may mask pain that would normally serve to warn you that you're overdoing it.
- Cool down.
- Be aware of warning signs including chest pain or tightness, dizziness or faintness, pain in an arm or your jaw, severe shortness of breath, an irregular heartbeat, excessive fatigue, severe joint or muscle pain, or joint swelling. If you experience any of these, stop immediately and seek medical attention.

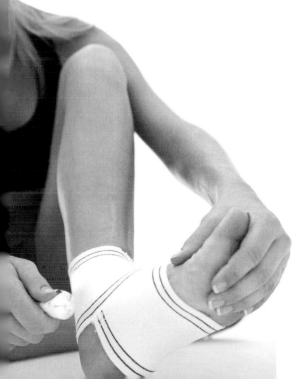

- Gradually increase the intensity of your activity. If you've been walking at a 15-minute-per-mile pace, step it up to 14 or 13. This is a particularly good strategy for strength training. Making your muscles work harder, rather than longer, is the best way to increase strength gains. Be careful to increase the intensity of your activity gradually. Adding too much at once can lead to pain and injury.
- Try interval training. Work out at varying intensities.
- Consider cross-training. Varying your activities can help you avoid plateaus, as can switching the order in which you do your exercises.

"Use it or lose it"

The beneficial effects of fitness are transitory — when you stop exercising, you'll begin to lose them. This use-it-or-lose-it effect is known as detraining. If you're laid up with an injury or take a break from exercise, some loss of fitness is inevitable. The good news is that you can take steps to avoid or minimize the loss.

How quickly detraining happens depends on how fit you were to begin with, how long you've been exercising and how long you've stopped. It also depends on what activities you were doing.

For cardiovascular activities, people who are extremely conditioned experience a rapid drop in fitness during the first three weeks of detraining, which then tapers off. People with low to moderate fitness levels show a more gradual, steady reduction. At any given point during detraining, a more fit person will maintain a higher level of fitness than will a less fit person.

Gains in strength from resistance or weight training may last longer. Newly gained strength may be retained for up to six weeks after you stop training, and you can retain about half the strength you gain for up to a year. Strength declines very slowly in muscle groups that are used regularly.

What's more, when you start strength training again, you'll return to your previous levels of strength with less effort. This is because of muscle memory — the learning that took place earlier.

Your ability to perform a specific sport or activity usually declines if you abandon the activity for an extended time. Some sport-specific skills, such as riding a bike, are easily maintained, while others, such as delivering a powerful and accurate serve in tennis, require well-trained muscles.

To avoid losing the health and fitness benefits you've worked so hard to achieve, cut back on exercise, if you need to, rather than cut it out altogether. If you can't do strength training three times a week, you can still maintain most of your gains by training once or twice a week. If you can't run, try walking, swimming or cycling instead. The most important thing is that you remain active.

Step 3
Eat Well

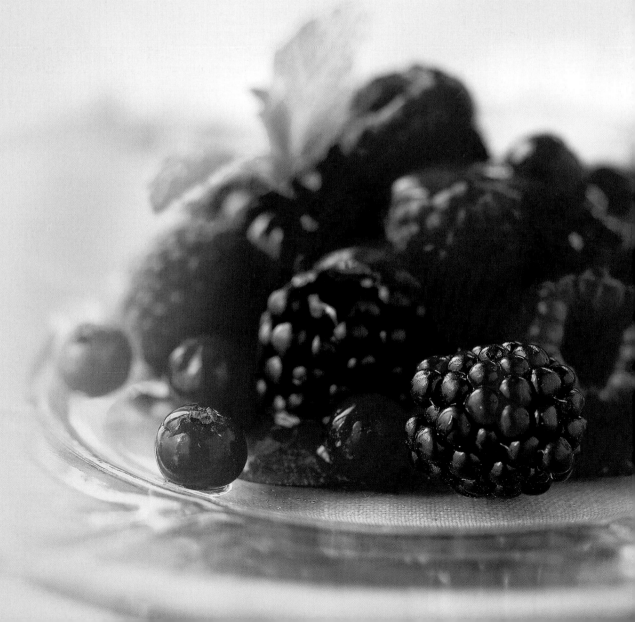

A visit with Jennifer Nelson

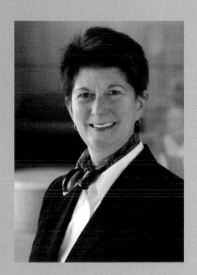

Jennifer Nelson, R.D.
Dietetics

Because food is so readily available, eating has become a continuous event. Unfortunately, most grab-and-go foods generally aren't ones that promote health. Years ago, we weren't just grabbing something right around the corner at the coffee machine. We'd have to walk somewhere or bring our lunch from home. And the types of foods that were available in the grocery store were whole foods — fruits and vegetables and fewer processed foods. You couple these changes with a more sedentary, high-stress lifestyle, and we've created an atmosphere where good nutrition choices must be part of a person's conscious decision making. Eating well can have a major impact on long-term health. And, a nutritious diet doesn't have to be dreary, complex and untasty.

You'll find that you can incorporate healthy eating into a busy lifestyle and do just fine. Plus, it can be fun and delicious! There are many options, and you don't need extensive cooking skills — just a few ideas and a spirit of creativity. You could put vegetables and chicken into a slow cooker and go to the soccer game, or make and pack peanut butter sandwiches on rustic whole-grain bread with crunchy apples. You can cook from scratch and have everything on the table in a half-hour, just like you would if you were pulling a convenience food out of a microwave. It's going to take a conscious effort to go back to the basics, but once you've done it a few times, it becomes a skill that you won't forget — that can save a lot of time, and your health!

Q: What is one simple thing I can do to noticeably improve my diet?

A: Try to include plant-based foods at every meal — vegetables, fruits and whole grains. There are three great benefits from eating more plant foods: First, they're great sources of health-enhancing vitamins, minerals, fiber and phytochemicals (natural chemicals found in plants that fight diseases). Second, plant-based foods are more filling and are also lower in calories and fat so they can help with weight control. Third, by making plant foods centerstage for your meals, you'll cut back on high-fat animal foods like meats, eggs and cheeses — foods that should be eaten in lean, low-fat versions and smaller amounts.

Q: Can I have an unhealthy diet if I'm not overweight?

A: Yes. Weight is determined by calories — one of the many nutrients that contribute to health. It's entirely possible to eat the right amount of calories, but the foods you choose can lack other essential nutrients and lead to health problems. For example, too little folate during pregnancy may cause birth defects. Too little calcium and vitamin D over time can contribute to osteoporosis. Make your calories count by choosing foods that are packed with nutrients.

Q: Can a healthy diet prevent cancer?

A: The American Cancer Society and the American Institute for Cancer Research agree that diet contributes significantly to various types of cancer — 30 percent to 40 percent of cancers are directly linked to dietary choices. You can reduce your cancer risk by eating a diet rich in a variety of vegetables, fruits, legumes and minimally processed grains. Limit high-fat foods, especially those from animal sources.

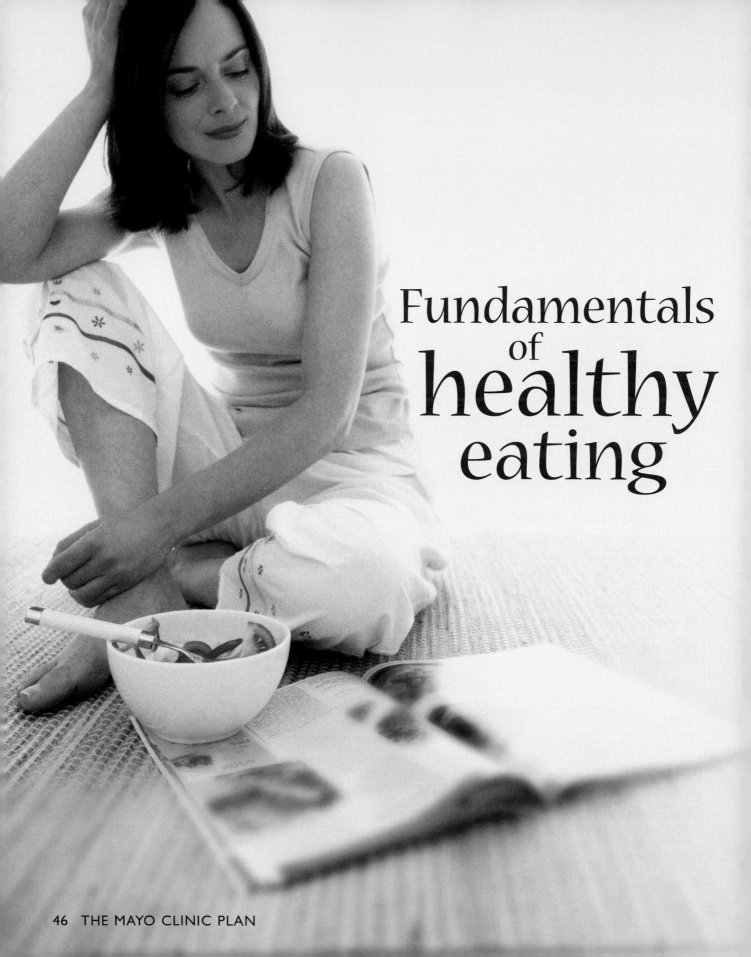

Fundamentals of healthy eating

O K, so if something tastes good, it can't be good for you, right? Wrong! Great taste and good health can and should go hand in hand. It's a point worth strongly emphasizing — food that's good for you can be deliciously rich in flavor. And perhaps just as important, it can be easy to plan for and prepare.

This section of *The Mayo Clinic Plan* helps you understand the basics of good nutrition, and how you can literally eat your way to better health.

What you eat does matter

Research has shown and clinical experience has confirmed that what you eat directly affects your health. An unhealthy diet high in saturated fat can lead to health problems ranging from cardiovascular disease to cancer. But cooking with nutritious ingredients — such as vegetables, fruits, and whole grains — may actually lower your risk of developing many diseases.

People who regularly enjoy meals made with a variety of healthy ingredients may lower their chances of developing heart disease, diabetes, many kinds of cancer, osteoporosis, obesity, age-related vision loss, digestive disorders, and more.

Flavor comes first

Although good food is crucial to good health, deciding to eat wisely doesn't mean having to seek out unusual "health foods" such as broccoli sprouts and wheatgrass. It doesn't mean denying yourself desserts and other delicacies you love. And it doesn't mean food that's complicated or expensive. After all, some of the world's most tempting dishes are built around the season's best produce, prepared simply to bring out the fullest flavors.

We enjoy an abundance of food choices unparalleled in history — just take a look around the aisles of a well-stocked supermarket. With so many great ingredients near at hand, it's quite easy to prepare dishes that not only are a pleasure to serve and eat but also are beneficial to your health.

The eating philosophy reflected in this book is to enjoy an extraordinary variety of foods that both taste terrific and are terrific for you.

A new philosophy of eating

The healthy eating approach outlined in this section is based on The Mayo Clinic Healthy Weight Pyramid (shown on page 54). The pyramid was designed to help people control their weight and improve their health. Its principles apply to anyone who simply wants to better his or her eating habits and health.

The pyramid focuses on a wide variety of foods that provide an array of valuable nutrients. It emphasizes foods that are low in energy density — that is, they're filling and satisfying but low in calories — so that you can eat well without feeling either guilty or deprived.

As you read on, you'll discover a whole new philosophy of cooking and eating, along with helpful suggestions on menu planning

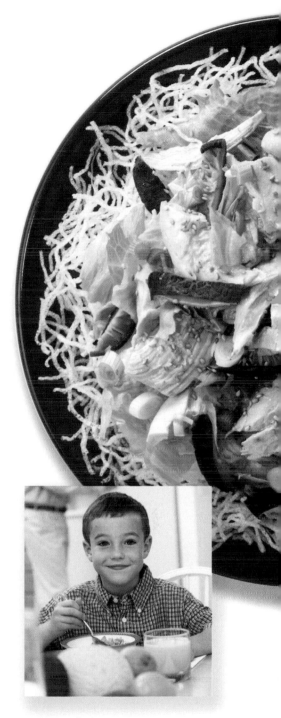

and practical insights on the ingredients themselves. Later in the book, we provide menus and recipes to help you get started. To eat well — and healthfully — just help yourself.

Nutrition nuggets

If you figure eating well means counting calories or tallying fat grams, it's time to think about food in a different manner. Eating well means enjoying great taste as well as great nutrition.

Because your body is a complex machine, it needs a variety of foods to achieve a balanced mix of energy. That variety — emphasizing vegetables, fruits and whole grains — can lead to a diet that provides a rich supply of nutrients, fiber and other substances associated with better health. In addition to these benefits, a variety of foods introduces you to myriad textures and flavors that boost your eating satisfaction and pleasure.

By learning more about how your body uses the nutrients different foods provide, you'll better understand how eating well affects your health.

Getting a good mix of nutrients

The food you eat supplies many types of nutrients, which provide the energy your body needs in order to grow and function. These nutrients include carbohydrates, fats, protein, vitamins and minerals. Food is also a source of water and fiber, and it provides disease-fighting compounds called phytochemicals.

Carbohydrates

Carbohydrates can be simple or complex. Simple carbohydrates are the sugars found in fruits, honey and milk. They're absorbed quickly into the body for energy. Complex carbohydrates, also known as starches, are found primarily in whole grains, pasta, potatoes, beans and vegetables. Digestion is required to change complex carbohydrates into simple sugars.

Complex carbohydrates in their natural state, such as whole-grain products, contain many vitamins and minerals and fiber. During processing, complex carbohydrates are refined, meaning most of the fiber and some nutrients have been removed.

Fats

Fats are a natural component of various foods, which come in different forms. Oils used in cooking are a form of fat. Fats are found in foods of animal origin, such as meat, dairy products, poultry and fish. You can also find fat in common plant foods such as nuts, olives and avocados. Some fats are better for you than others.

Protein

Protein builds and repairs body structures, carries nutrients to your cells, produces body chemicals and regulates processes.

Adequate protein is critical, but when you eat more protein than needed, the extra protein is converted into body fat. You can get protein from a variety of sources. Legumes, poultry, seafood, lean meat, dairy products, nuts and seeds are your richest sources of protein.

Do you need a calcium supplement?

Calcium is a mineral important for strong teeth and bones and for muscle and nerve function. Sufficient amounts of calcium in your diet greatly reduce your risk of osteoporosis.

The recommended daily intake of calcium is 1,000 to 1,200 milligrams (mg) for adults. Unfortunately, many adults don't consume enough calcium. If you're trying to lose weight, you may need to monitor calcium intake because of reduced calorie consumption.

To help reach your calcium goal, consider eating more low-fat dairy products and dark green vegetables such as broccoli. Some cereals, breads and juices may contain added calcium. You may also consider taking a calcium supplement. If you're unsure whether you're getting adequate calcium, talk with your doctor or a registered dietitian.

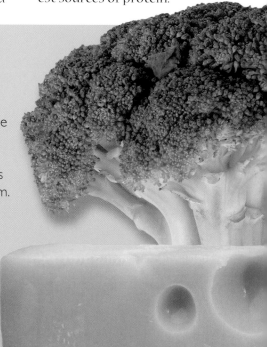

Vitamins

Vitamins help your body process carbohydrates, fats and protein. They also help produce blood cells, hormones and genetic material, as well as chemicals for the nervous system. Vitamin deficiencies lead to various diseases. Eating a variety of foods helps ensure you get all of the vitamins you need.

Minerals

Minerals such as calcium, magnesium and phosphorus are important to the health of your bones and teeth. Sodium, potassium and chloride, commonly referred to as electrolytes, help regulate the water and chemical balance in your body. Your body needs smaller amounts of minerals such as iron, iodine, zinc, copper, fluoride, selenium and manganese, commonly referred to as trace minerals. All have unique roles in ensuring good health.

Water

It's easy to take water for granted, but it's a vital nutritional requirement. Many foods, especially fruit, contain a lot of water. The most direct way to get water into your system is to drink it. Water plays a role in many major body functions. It regulates body temperature, carries nutrients and oxygen to cells via the bloodstream and helps carry away waste. Water also helps cushion joints and protects organs and tissues.

Fiber

Fiber is the part of plant foods that your body doesn't absorb. The two main types of fiber are soluble and insoluble, and fiber-rich foods usually contain both. Foods high in soluble fiber include citrus fruits, strawberries, apples, legumes, oatmeal and oat bran.

Soluble fiber helps lower blood cholesterol and adds bulk to stools. Insoluble fiber is found in many vegetables, wheat bran, and whole-grain breads, pasta and cereals. Insoluble fiber stimulates the gastrointestinal tract, helping to prevent constipation.

Phytochemicals

Many of these chemical compounds found in plants have antioxidant properties. Others help optimize cell functions. Phytochemicals help prevent chronic diseases such as cardiovascular disease, cancer and diabetes. Examples include flavonoids found in fruits, vegetables and tea; isoflavones found in soy products, beans and legumes; phytosterols found in nuts, seeds, whole grains and plant oils; and carotenoids — such as beta carotene, lycopene and lutein —present in red and yellow vegetables.

Where calories come from

Calories are used to measure any kind of energy, but people most often associate the term *calorie* with nutrition.

Carbohydrates, fats and protein are the types of nutrients that contain calories and thus are the main energy sources for your body. The amount of energy each nutrient provides varies, as well as the mechanism by which the energy is supplied. Alcohol also contains calories. *Empty calories* is a term often applied to alcohol, as well as sugar. They contribute calories, but no other essential nutrients.

Carbohydrates are the nutrients in the food you eat that get used up first. During digestion, they're released into your bloodstream and converted into glucose, or blood sugar. When there's an energy demand, the glucose is absorbed immediately into your body's cells to provide energy. If there's no immediate demand, glucose can be stored in your liver and muscles. When these storage sites become full, excess glucose is converted into fatty acids and stored in fat tissue for later use.

Fats are an extremely concentrated form of energy and they pack the most calories. When digested, they're broken down into fatty acids, which can be used immediately for energy or for other body processes. If there's an excess of fatty acids, a small quantity can be stored in your muscles, but most of them are stored in fat tissue. There's virtually no limit to how much fat your body can store.

Protein has many responsibilities in your body, including supplying energy for physical activity if your body runs out of calories. This can happen if you consume too few calories or are involved in prolonged physical activity. Excess calories from protein are stored in fat tissue.

Vitamins, minerals, water and fiber don't contain calories. Although these nutrients may not provide energy, they're still vital to your health and well-being. When they're lacking from your diet, you increase your risk of serious illness. Other substances in food, such as cholesterol, also don't provide calories.

Your energy account

Imagine that the energy needs of your body are like a bank account. Lots of transactions go on in this account. You have daily deposits, and you have daily withdrawals. Your deposits are food, with three nutrients providing the bulk of your energy: carbohydrates, fats and protein. When you eat, you're adding to your energy account — in the form of calories.

Withdrawals on this account can be made in three basic ways, each of which burns calories. The most obvious type of withdrawal is when you exert yourself by doing physical activity. Energy spent doing

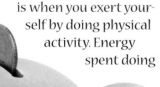

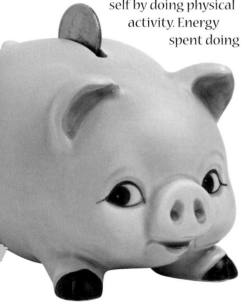

physical activity is variable. It can be as low as 100 calories a day for inactive people and higher than 3,000 calories a day for very active people.

A second way your body withdraws energy is to meet your basic needs, including breathing, blood circulation and maintaining body temperature. Even when you're at rest, your body is using energy. Energy use at rest is commonly called basal metabolic rate (BMR). Your BMR accounts for one-half to two-thirds of your total energy expenditure.

The third way you burn calories is when you digest, absorb and process food. This accounts for about 10 percent of your energy expenditure. The energy needs of your BMR and for digestion remain relatively steady and aren't easy to change. The best way to increase your energy withdrawal — in other words, to burn more calories — is to increase your physical activity.

Influences on your energy account

If everyone were physically and functionally identical, it would be easy to determine energy needs for all kinds of activity. But other factors affect your energy account. People differ in many ways, and their energy needs vary accordingly. Some of the factors that influence your BMR and your overall energy needs are age, body size and composition, and sex.

Age
Children and adolescents, who are in the process of developing their bones, muscles and tissues, need more calories per pound

Food sources of energy

Fats supply more calories per gram than do carbohydrates and proteins combined. Alcohol has calories, too.

Nutrient	Calories (per gram)
Fats	9
Alcohol	7
Carbohydrates	4
Protein	4

than do adults. In fact, infants need the most calories per pound of any age group because of their rapid growth and development. As hormone levels and body composition change with age, so does a person's basal metabolic rate. By the time you reach adulthood, your BMR and energy needs are declining, generally at a rate of 2 percent a decade.

Body size and composition
In order to function properly, a bigger body mass requires more energy, and thus more calories, than does a smaller body mass. In addition, muscle burns more calories than fat does, so the more muscle you have in relation to fat, the higher your BMR. Based on this principle, you can slightly increase your BMR and the amount of energy you burn by building up your muscle mass through regular physical activity.

Sex
Men usually have less body fat and more muscle than do

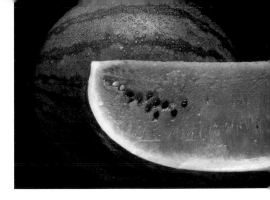

women of the same age and weight. This is why men generally have a higher resting energy expenditure and higher energy requirements than do women.

Balancing your account

Your body weight is a reflection of your energy account. Daily fluctuations of your weight indicate the daily changes in your account.

If you withdraw from the account approximately the same amount of energy as you deposit, your weight stays the same. If you expend more from the account than you deposit, you lose weight.

There's an important number in this energy equation. Because 1 pound of body fat contains 3,500 calories, you'd need to consume 3,500 excess calories to gain a pound, and conversely, you'd need to burn 3,500 calories more than you take in to lose a pound. This knowledge may seem impractical on a daily basis, but it does generally indicate what it takes to gain, lose or maintain your weight.

Many people prefer keeping their energy accounts balanced — meaning there's just enough calories in the accounts to meet their energy needs but no more. The tricky part is that energy needs vary from day to day. The amount of food that people eat also varies. Therefore, the balance between calories consumed and calories expended is constantly shifting.

Tracking these shifts would require a bit of old-fashioned accounting — tallying up all the sources of energy income (consumption of calories) and all the forms of energy expenditure — including your BMR and your energy needs for digestion. Who has the time and resources to make this daily effort?

Instead, you can maintain a healthy balance of calories consumed and calories expended by eating the right mix of foods and making sure that you include enough physical activity in your day. In the next chapter, we discuss what foods you should eat the most of and the number of foods servings you should aim for to maintain your current weight or to lose weight, while still ensuring your diet is providing you adequate nutrition.

It's not solely the kinds of food you eat that make you gain weight. Equally important are the amounts of food you consume and how active you are. True, you can eat any food you like and maintain or lose weight as long as your total caloric consumption is equal to or less than the total calories burned. But a diet built on nutritious foods is best — for many good reasons.

Ensuring good health

To eat healthy, it's important not to focus only on foods that are lower in calories. You also want to make sure to include in your diet foods that are rich in a variety of nutrients.

Heart and blood vessel (cardiovascular) disease, high blood pressure and many cancers are linked most notably to being overweight and eating foods high in saturated fat.

If, for example, the bulk of your diet consists of foods that contain considerable saturated fat, such as red meat, bacon or butter, you run the risk of increasing your low-density lipoprotein (LDL, or "bad") cholesterol level, narrowing your arteries and restricting blood flow, which could potentially result in a heart attack.

Evidence also links a diet that consists mainly of highly processed foods and very few vegetables, fruits and whole grains to conditions such as diabetes, some cancers and cardiovascular disease.

In addition, if you aren't getting enough vegetables and fruits in your diet, you're missing many vital health benefits. Vegetables and fruits contain:

- Numerous vitamins and minerals needed to ensure proper functioning of vital body processes, and to ward off disease
- Phytochemicals, a group of compounds that may help prevent chronic diseases, such as cardiovascular disease and diabetes, and cancer
- Antioxidants, substances that slow down oxidation, a natural process that leads to cell and tissue damage

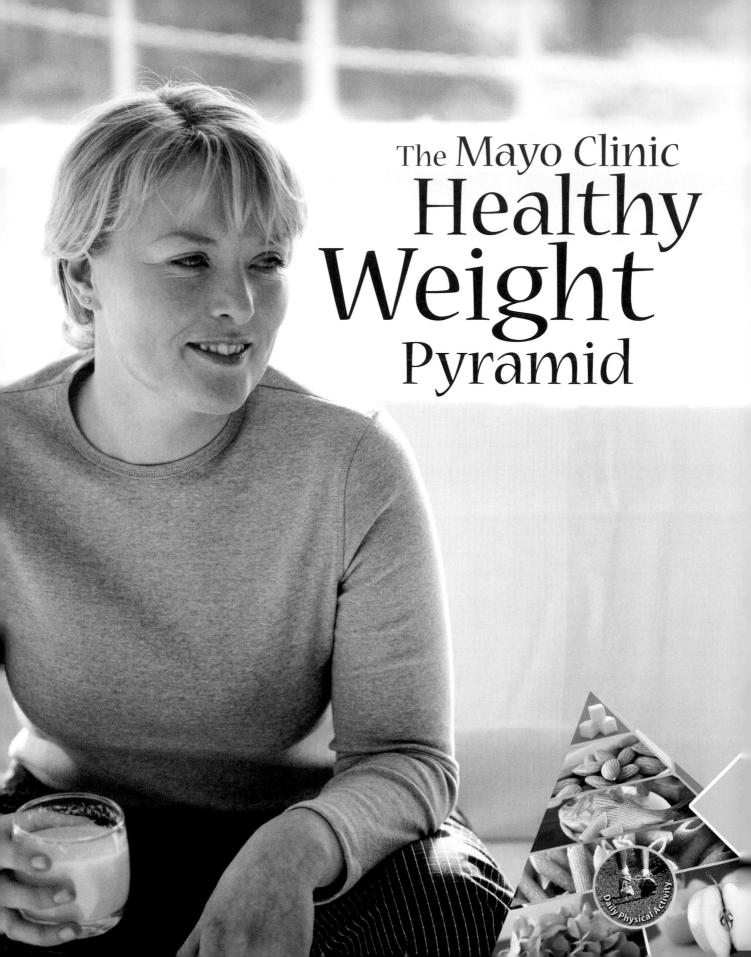

The Mayo Clinic
Healthy
Weight
Pyramid

To eat well and maintain a healthy weight over your lifetime, it's important that you adopt an eating plan that you enjoy and never tire of. That means no severe restrictions on the foods you can eat and no extreme hunger. Your daily diet should include a wide variety of foods, and it should include enough food to fill you up at meals so that you don't become hungry an hour or two after you're done eating.

The Mayo Clinic Healthy Weight Pyramid can help you achieve these goals. The pyramid is an easy-to-use guide to what you need to eat each day from the six food groups to achieve good nutrition and maintain a healthy weight.

Energy density

The Mayo Clinic Healthy Weight Pyramid is based on the concept of energy density. To maintain your body weight, the amount of energy you take in (calories consumed) must equal the amount of energy you expend (calories burned). To lose weight, you need to create an energy deficit, by decreasing your energy intake or increasing your energy expenditure. Most commonly you need to do both.

Think volume

All foods contain a certain number of calories in a given amount (volume). Foods that contain many calories in a small portion are described as high in energy density. These include most high-fat foods, simple sugars, alcohol, fast foods, sodas, candies and processed foods.

Foods such as vegetables and fruits have fewer calories in a greater volume. These types of foods are considered low in energy density.

Two primary factors play important roles in what makes food less energy dense and more filling: water and fiber.

- **Water.** Most fruits and vegetables contain a lot of water, which provides volume and weight to what you eat but not calories.
- **Fiber.** The high fiber content in foods such as vegetables, fruits and whole grains provides bulk to your diet, so it makes you feel full sooner. Fiber also takes longer to digest, making you feel full for a longer period of time.

The idea that you can feel full on fewer calories may sound like one of those diet gimmicks. But the energy density concept makes sense. Research suggests that feeling full is strongly determined by the volume and weight of food in your stomach, not necessarily by the amount of calories you eat. By choosing foods with a low energy density, you can consume fewer calories while eating similar amounts of food as you did before.

Researchers at Mayo Clinic and elsewhere have tested the concept of energy density. Participants in several studies who switched to a diet containing low-energy-density foods were able to lose significant amounts of weight. More importantly, they were able to keep a good deal of the weight off over time, decreasing their risk of weight-related diseases.

The food groups

The six food groups that make up the Mayo Clinic Healthy Weight Pyramid are vegetables, fruits, carbohydrates, protein and dairy, fats, and sweets.

Most of the foods we eat fit into one of these groups. But no matter how you attempt to organize them, foods don't fall neatly into categories. The food groups within The Mayo Clinic Healthy Weight Pyramid were organized based on these factors:

- The groups differ in their levels of energy density — foods with the lowest energy density are at the pyramid base.
- The foods in each group share common health benefits.
- The breakdown is practical in terms of your ability to select and prepare different meals.

What's different?

Some main differences between The Mayo Clinic Healthy Weight Pyramid and other food pyramids are that the Mayo pyramid:

- Is geared to maintaining weight as well as losing weight
- Has the vegetable and fruit groups as the base
- Incorporates and unlimited allowance of fresh vegetables and fruit
- Emphasizes health-promoting choices within each food group

Energy density

All foods have a certain number of calories within a given amount (volume). Some foods, such as desserts and processed foods, are high in energy density, meaning they contain a large number of calories within just a small portion. Other foods, such as vegetables, fruits and whole-grain products, are low in energy density, meaning a large portion contains only a few calories. By eating foods low in energy density, you get more food, consume fewer calories and still walk away from the table feeling full. The food on each of the platters to the right equals 1,200 calories. As you can see, butter, which is high in energy density, provides just a small portion of food for those calories. Green peppers and lettuce, on the other hand, are low in energy density, so you get a lot more food for the calories.

THE MAYO CLINIC HEALTHY WEIGHT PYRAMID

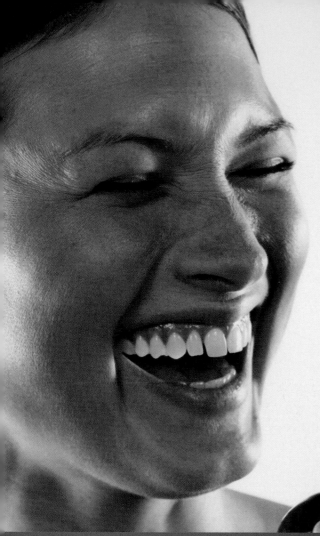

The Mayo Clinic Healthy Weight Pyramid is your guide to achieving and maintaining a healthy weight. Its triangular shape shows you where to focus your attention when selecting healthy foods. You want to eat more from the food groups at the base of the pyramid and less from those at the top. The number of servings you should consume from each food group is based on your daily calorie goals.

Starting calorie goals

SWEETS

FATS

PROTEIN/DAIRY

CARBOHYDRATES

Daily Physical Activity

FRUITS

VEGETABLES

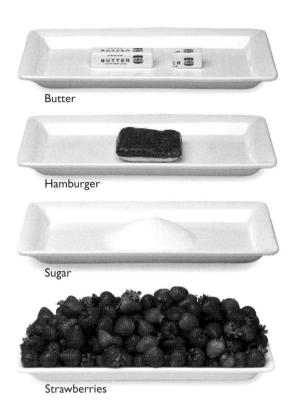

Butter

Hamburger

Sugar

Strawberries

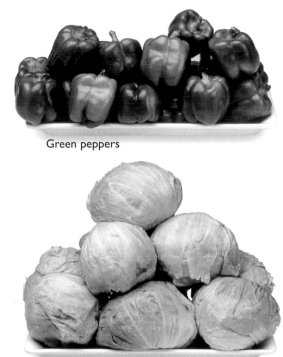

Green peppers

Lettuce

Daily serving recommendations for various calorie levels				
1,200	1,400	1,600	1,800	2,000
Up to 75 calories daily				
3	3	3	4	5
3	4	5	6	7
4	5	6	7	8
3 or more	4 or more	5 or more ▶		
4 or more	4 or more	5 or more ▶		

Vegetables and fruits

It's hardly news that vegetables and fruits are good for you. The real news is why. More and more is being learned about how fresh produce, beyond its rich stores of vitamins, can supply us with substances that help ward off many illnesses.

Strong evidence continues to show that people who regularly eat generous helpings of a variety of vegetables run a lower risk of developing the leading killers of American adults: cardiovascular disease, high blood pressure, cancer and diabetes.

Most vegetables are loaded with vitamins, and they contain the antioxidants beta carotene and vitamin C. Antioxidants are thought to help inhibit molecules called oxygen free radicals, which can damage healthy cells. Vegetables are also key sources of essential minerals, including potassium and magnesium, important in the control of blood pressure. Many are rich in health-enhancing fiber, and some even have calcium.

In addition, researchers have identified another class of substances in these plants — called phytochemicals — that appear to offer some protection against cancer. Tomatoes, for instance, get their red color from lycopene. Studies suggest that getting plenty of this phytochemical may lower prostate cancer risk.

Like many vegetables, fruits also have an abundance of fiber — not to mention a long list of healthful antioxidants, including vitamin C. Researchers have also discovered that many fruits contain generous amounts of flavonoids, substances that apparently work together to lower the risk of cancer and heart disease. Some fruits and vegetables contain the antioxidants lutein and zeaxanthin, which may help guard against certain conditions related to aging, such as the eye disease macular degeneration. Tree nuts, for instance, are rich in a little-known compound called beta-sitosterol, which is believed to help lower blood cholesterol.

These many benefits are the reason why under the pyramid there's no limit on the daily servings of fresh and frozen vegetables and fruits. The exceptions are dried fruits and fruit juices, which measure for measure are much higher in calories than the fresh fruits from which they're made.

THE GOAL (based on 1,200 daily calories): four or more vegetable and three or more fruit servings a day. A vegetable serving is about 25 calories; a fruit serving, 60 calories.

GETTING THERE:

A day's menu might include (each item is 1 serving)

1 tomato or 8 cherry tomatoes
2 cups (2 oz.) salad greens
½ cup (2 oz.) carrot sticks
1 cup (5 oz.) broccoli
1 orange, apple or banana
½ grapefruit
1 cup (3 oz.) grapes
1 cup (4 oz.) berries

Snack suggestions

- Make a fruit smoothie by blending fruit with low-fat yogurt or skim milk.

- Cut fruit in slices or halves and dip the pieces in low-fat cottage cheese or yogurt.

- Make frozen fruit chips. Purée or crush fruit and then freeze it.

- Freeze fresh grapes and enjoy them when the weather is warm.

- Use chunks of fresh fruit to make fruit kebabs on skewers.

- Dip partially cooked vegetables (carrots, green beans, broccoli, cauliflower) in cottage cheese, hummus, low-fat ranch dressing or yogurt dip.

- Place a light coat of peanut butter or low-fat cream cheese on bell pepper slices, zucchini chunks or tomato wedges.

- Spread peanut butter on celery slices and top the peanut butter with raisins.

- Mix low-fat ricotta cheese with unsweetened pineapple and spread on celery or green pepper strips.

- Make vegetable kebabs with bell pepper strips, mushrooms, cherry tomatoes and zucchini chunks.

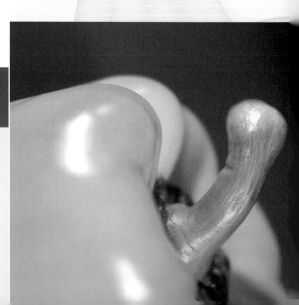

10 ways to eat more vegetables and fruits

Fresh vegetables and fruits are the foundation of a healthy diet and successful weight loss. However, for some people, making sure they have a few servings of vegetables and fruits in their diets every day is a struggle. Here are tips that might help change that:

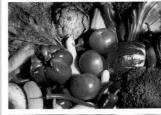
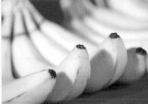
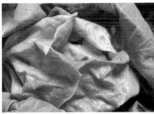
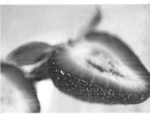

- Add a banana, strawberries or another favorite fruit to your cereal or yogurt at breakfast.

- Include a small salad with one of your main meals of the day.

- When eating a full meal, work on your vegetable portions right away, rather than reserving them for the end after you've finished other items.

- Stir-fry vegetables with a small portion of poultry, seafood or meat.

- Use fresh fruit and fruit sauces as toppings on desserts and pancakes.

- When you're in a hurry, have ready-to-eat frozen vegetables handy as a quick addition to a meal. Use fresh vegetables and fruits that require little preparation, such as baby carrots, cherry tomatoes, broccoli, cauliflower, grapes and apples.

- Liven up your sandwiches with vegetables such as tomato, lettuce, onion, peppers and cucumber.

- When you have a craving for chips, have a small handful with lots of fresh salsa.

- For dessert, have baked apples, grilled pineapple or a bowl of berries.

- Experimenting with new tastes keeps you challenged. Try vegetables and fruits that you're unfamiliar with, perhaps mango, papaya, tomatillo, jicama and star fruit, which can be obtained at most grocery stores or specialty food stores.

What if I don't like vegetables and fruits?

Some people find vegetables and fruits to be bland and boring. A common opinion is that vegetables and fruits don't have much taste, or that they all taste the same. Not true. Vegetables and fruits can be tasty — you just have to know which ones to eat, or how to prepare them. Much of what you eat is conditioned — that is, over time, you've learned to like it.

In the same respect, you can learn to like new foods, such as vegetables and fruits. To learn to like vegetables and fruits, you can experiment. Here are some suggestions.

- Keep in mind that you don't need to like all vegetables and fruits, just some.

- Instead of the familiar apples and oranges, buy fresh fruits that you haven't tried before, perhaps kiwi, mango, Bing cherries and apricots.

- Try different ways of preparation. For example, grill pineapple or make fruit smoothies.

- If you don't care for raw vegetables, lightly cook them and see if you prefer them with a softer texture. Sprinkle them with herbs for flavor.

- To get more vegetables and fruits into your diet, incorporate them with other foods or recipes: Add vegetables to a favorite soup, replace some of the hamburger in casseroles with chopped vegetables, add peppers and onions to your pizza, include fresh fruit with your morning cereal, stir fruit in with yogurt or cottage cheese.

Carbohydrates

Think of every kind of food containing carbohydrates laid out in a line. At one end are whole wheat, oats and brown rice. In the middle sit white flour, white rice, potatoes and pastas. And at the far end are cookies, candies and soft drinks.

The foods in that spectrum incorporate all three kinds of carbohydrates: fiber, starch and sugar. It's not hard to point to the healthy and less healthy ends — unrefined whole grains on one hand, refined sugar on the other.

But the health pros and cons of many items in the middle aren't so clear. Rice, pasta, bread and potatoes can all shift depending on how they're produced and served.

Consider, for example, white and whole-wheat (whole-meal) breads. Both begin as whole grains, as do both white and brown rice. That whole, or unrefined, grain consists of outer layers, known as the bran and germ, surrounding a starchy interior, called the endosperm.

Whole grains abound with vitamins, minerals and other important nutrients. Some whole grains contain estrogen-like substances that may help protect against some forms of cancer.

During processing, however, the bran and germ are refined, and by the time the wheat has become a loaf of white bread or the rice is a steaming white side dish, the grains have lost many of their natural vitamins and almost all of their fiber — just as the edible skins people often remove from potatoes are full of nutrients and fiber. That's why it's wise to choose whole-grain breads, pastas and cereals whenever you can, and to serve brown rice instead of white. In addition, unprocessed foods retain many of their phytochemicals.

Of course, many foods not always thought of as carbohydrates contain amounts of fiber, starch and sugar — not only vegetables and fruits but also sweets, chips and other processed products.

The key word to remember here is *whole*. Generally, the message is that simple: The less refined a carbohydrate food, the better it is for you.

Fitting more fiber into your day

Grains, fruits and vegetables all contain a kind of carbohydrate, called fiber, that resists digestive enzymes and cannot be absorbed by your body. There are two main types — insoluble and soluble — both of which are found in varying amounts in most plants.

Fiber-rich foods slow the uptake of glucose, thus helping to keep blood sugar steady. Research suggests that the more fiber people get from grains, the lower their risk of type 2 diabetes. Experts recommend consuming 21 to 38 grams of fiber a day.

- Insoluble fiber — called roughage — is coarse, indigestible plant material best known for promoting healthy digestion. Many common vegetables and whole grains contain significant amounts.

- Soluble fiber — vegetable matter that turns goopy in water — helps lower blood cholesterol levels. Barley, oats, and beans contain notable amounts.

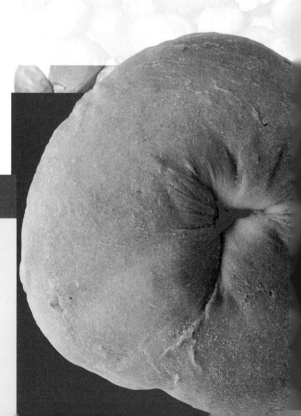

THE GOAL: four carbohydrate servings a day, mostly whole grains. A carbohydrate serving is about 70 calories.

GETTING THERE:

A day's menu might include (each item is 1 serving)
½ cup (1½ oz.) dry cereal
½ whole-grain English muffin
1 slice whole-grain bread
½ cup (3 oz.) cooked bulgur

2 cups (½ oz.) fat-free popcorn
½ cup (3 oz.) cooked whole-wheat pasta
½ large baked sweet potato
30 pretzel sticks

Carbs: Setting the record straight

Carbohydrates don't make you fat; excess calories do. Recently, many diets have promoted eating low-carbohydrate foods as a way to lose weight. These diets claim that carbohydrates stimulate insulin secretion, which promotes body fat. So, the logic goes, reducing carbohydrates will reduce body fat.

As a matter of fact, carbohydrates do stimulate insulin secretion immediately after they're consumed, but this is a normal process that allows carbohydrates to be absorbed into cells. People who gain weight on high-carbohydrate diets do so because they're eating excess calories. Excess calories from any source — whether it contains a lot of carbohydrates or only a few — will cause weight gain.

Furthermore, some low-carbohydrate diets restrict grains, fruits and vegetables and emphasize the consumption of protein and dairy products, which can be high calorie and loaded with saturated fat and cholesterol. Plant-based foods not only are low in saturated fat and cholesterol-free but also are loaded with vitamins, minerals and other nutrients. These nutrients play a protective role in fighting serious diseases such as cancer, osteoporosis, high blood pressure and heart disease.

So, be skeptical of the low-carbohydrate claims. Many carbohydrate-containing foods are healthy and they can be an important part of a weight-loss plan, but they should be eaten as part of a well-balanced diet.

Is eating sugar unhealthy?

Sugar isn't necessarily bad, but most sugars provide only calories and little nutritional value. Sugars are simple carbohydrates. Sources include table sugar (sucrose), fruits and juices (fructose), and milk and milk products (lactose). Natural sources of sugar are generally slightly better for you than foods with lots of added, refined sugar. Refined sugar has a high energy density.

Current U.S. Department of Agriculture Dietary Guidelines for Americans offer the following recommendations:

- Limit your intake of beverages and foods that have simple sugars added during processing — not foods such as fruit and milk, which have natural sugar in them. Don't let soft drinks or other sweets crowd out other foods needed for health, such as water or low-fat milk and milk products.

- Check the food label before you buy. The ingredients list tells you what's in the food, including any sugar that has been added. Ingredients are listed in descending order by weight. In addition to the word *sugar* on the labels of many products, look for these lesser known ingredients, which are actually forms of simple sugar: corn syrup or sweetener, dextrose, high-fructose corn syrup and maltose. A food is likely to be high in added sugar content if these ingredients appear first or second in the ingredients list.

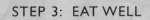

Protein and dairy

Protein is essential to human life. Your skin, bone, muscle and organ tissues are made up of protein, and its present in your blood, too. Protein is also found in foods, many of animal origin.

But despite what you may have heard, it's not necessary or even desirable to eat meat every day. Although rich in protein, many cuts of chicken, turkey, beef, lamb and pork are too high in saturated fat and cholesterol to include regularly for good health. Remember, other everyday ingredients, including low-fat dairy products, seafood and many plant foods, furnish protein, too.

Legumes — namely beans, lentils and peas — are also an excellent source. And because they have no cholesterol and very little fat, they're great for filling out or replacing dishes made with poultry or meat.

Unlike meat, beans actually help reduce low-density lipoprotein (LDL or "bad") cholesterol, and the minerals they contain help control blood pressure.

You may have heard that beans' protein is "incomplete," meaning it lacks essential amino acids that meats provide. That's true; among legumes, only soybeans have protein containing all the amino acids. However, the missing nutrients are plentiful in other plant foods, so people who lighten up on meat can easily get all the essential amino acids they need.

Likewise, fat-free and low-fat dairy products, especially milk and yogurt, can help supply you with protein. On top of that, milk is rich in calcium and is fortified with vitamin D, which helps bodies absorb that important bone-building mineral.

And don't neglect fish and shellfish. Not only are they fine protein sources, but some supply omega-3 fatty acids. Research suggests that most people would benefit by eating at least two servings of fish a week.

The omega-3 fatty acids in fish help lower triglycerides, fat particles in the blood that appear to raise your risk of cardiovascular disease. And they may also help prevent dangerous heartbeat disturbances known as arrhythmias, as well as help regulate blood pressure and improve immune function.

THE GOAL: three low-fat protein and dairy servings a day. A protein serving is about 110 calories.

GETTING THERE:

A day's menu might include (each item is 1 serving)

1 cup (8 fl. oz.) fat-free milk
1 cup (8 oz.) fat-free yogurt
¼ cup (1¼ oz.) feta cheese
½ cup (4 oz.) tofu
1½ oz. lean beef
3 oz. fish
½ cup (3 oz.) cooked beans
2½ oz. skinless chicken

Legume basics

Legumes, which include a variety of beans, peas and lentils, among others, are high in protein and make an excellent substitute for animal sources of protein.

Common types of legumes include white and navy beans, lima beans, pinto and black beans, black-eyed peas, split peas, brown and red lentils, and chickpeas (garbanzos).

Here are tips to help you select and store legumes, along with suggestions for different ways to serve legumes:

- Select legumes with a deep, almost glossy color. Dry-looking or faded legumes may have been stored for a long time and not taste as fresh.

- Look for legumes of a uniform size and condition. Similar-sized legumes cook more evenly. Check that the legumes are free of mold and aren't broken or cracked.

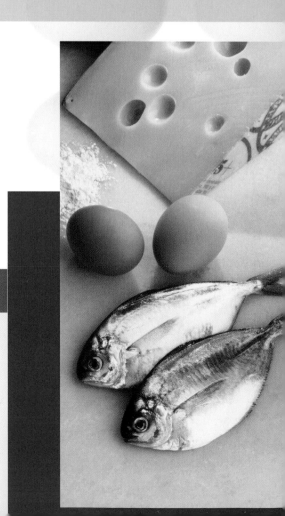

- Place dried legumes away from heat, light and moisture after purchase. They keep well for up to one year in an airtight container.

- Keep canned legumes such as beans in a cool, dry place. They safely store for two to five years.

- Sort and rinse legumes carefully before use. Bags of legumes may include a few small stones, fibers or misshapen or discolored items. Remove these before cooking.

- Soak most dried legumes before cooking. Beans and other large, dried legumes require soaking in room temperature water overnight, a step that rehydrates them for more even cooking. Split peas and lentils don't require soaking.

- Use canned legumes for convenience. Rinse them to remove any sodium added during processing.

- Legumes are great in soup. Find recipes for bean, lentil and split pea soups. When you don't have enough time to make your own, purchase soups that contain legumes. Also look for soups that are loaded with vegetables.

- Add legumes to casseroles. You can substitute legumes for hamburger or another type of meat. You can also add black beans or chickpeas (garbanzos) to salads.

- The main ingredient in hummus is chickpeas. You can make your own hummus or purchase it. Commercially prepared varieties of hummus are nutritionally similar to homemade. They often come seasoned in a variety of ways — scallion, garlic, red pepper, dill.

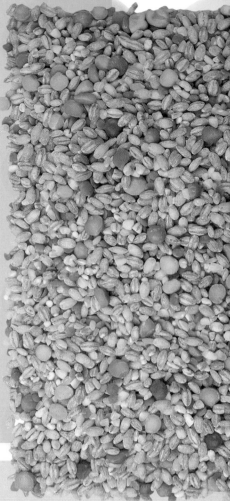

Fish facts

Like many people, you may be wondering which advice to take: Eat more fish because of the heart-healthy benefits of omega-3 fatty acids, or limit fish because of the risk of toxins, such as mercury. Toss in questions about farm-raised fish versus wild fish, and the issue becomes even cloudier.

What are the health benefits of eating fish?

Fish is generally low in calories, saturated fat and cholesterol, making it a good overall substitute for poultry and meat. It's also a good source of protein. Some types of fish, particularly fatty, cold-water fish, such as salmon, mackerel and herring, are also high in omega-3 fatty acids — a type of fat that helps protect against cardiovascular disease.

What are the health risks of eating fish?

As good as fish are for your health, be aware of potential downsides. Some types of fish may contain significant amounts of contaminants, such as mercury, polychlorinated biphenyls (PCBs), dioxins or other chemical pollutants. Fish acquire these toxins from water pollutants.

The major contaminate found in fish is mercury, which occurs naturally in trace amounts in the environment. But industrial pollution can produce mercury that accumulates in lakes, rivers and oceans. Large, predatory fish, such as shark, swordfish, king mackerel and tilefish, tend to have higher levels of mercury than do smaller fish.

If you eat fish that contains mercury, the toxin can accumulate in your body. Mercury is particularly harmful to brain and nervous system development of an unborn or young child. For this reason, women who are pregnant or trying to become pregnant, nursing mothers and young children should avoid all fish mentioned above and limit fish consumption to 12 ounces a week.

Individual states often issue advisories on how much fish caught in the state is safe to eat.

On average, though, the fish you buy at the store is safe to eat. Fish is an important part of a healthy diet, and it's recommended that you eat fish twice a week.

Fats

The idea that all fat is bad is so widespread that many people are surprised to hear health experts say some kinds can be beneficial. Studies over the past two decades have confirmed that people who replace much of the animal fat in their meals with liquid vegetable oils stand a good chance of bringing down their blood cholesterol levels, thereby lowering their risk of cardiovascular disease.

Other findings suggest that people who favor foods made with liquid oils, such as canola and olive oils, over ones with solid shortenings and margarines may derive similar health benefits.

Meats, seafood and many dairy products can be fatty, which is to say that some foods traditionally considered proteins can add significant fat to a day's meals. The Mayo Clinic Healthy Weight Pyramid recommends that you choose low-fat and lean versions of these foods.

The pyramid's fats section addresses only the high-fat ingredients that are typically added to a day's meals. These include salad dressings, cooking oils, butter and high-fat plant foods, such as avocado, olives, seeds and nuts. You want to limit fat servings to three daily and to choose fats that are healthy.

Not all fats are bad for you. Nuts, for instance, contain a type of oil that helps keep hearts and arteries free of harmful deposits. They also deliver many other key nutrients, including protein, thiamin, niacin, folate, selenium and vitamin E.

But while nuts, and products such as vegetable oils, may be beneficial, they're best used in moderation. A tablespoon of peanut butter weighs in at nearly 100 calories; a tablespoon of olive oil, 140. In other words, the goal is to use just enough of these naturally high-fat ingredients, but not too much.

Other fats are best kept to a minimum. Saturated fat, largely found in foods of animal origin, has long been known to raise low-density lipoprotein (LDL or "bad") cholesterol and lower high-density lipoprotein (HDL or "good") cholesterol. Research also has shown that foods high in trans fats, common in processed foods, have a similar impact on cholesterol levels.

THE GOAL: three fat servings a day. A fat serving is about 45 calories.

GETTING THERE:

A day's menu might include (each item is 1 serving)

7 almonds
4 walnut or pecan halves
1 ½ teaspoons peanut butter

1 tablespoon sunflower seeds
9 large olives
4 tablespoons fat-free mayonnaise
1 teaspoon canola or olive oil

Fats: Healthful and harmful

Easy does it

Eating wisely used to mean cutting back on all fat, but health experts now believe that some varieties of fat, used lightly, can actually be beneficial.

- Monounsaturates, in nuts, avocados, canola oil and olive oil, help lower blood levels of LDL cholesterol, a cause of heart attacks and strokes. They also help keep arteries clear by maintaining levels of helpful HDL cholesterol.

- Polyunsaturates, including corn and soy oils, also keep harmful LDL cholesterol levels down. Among them are the heart-healthy omega-3 fatty acids in fish, flaxseed, soybeans, tofu, walnuts, and walnut oil.

- Saturated fats, from meats, full-fat dairy products and tropical oils, raise blood levels of LDL cholesterol. Limit these fats by choosing low-fat dairy products and by combining lean meats with vegetables and grains.

- Trans fats, found in hydrogenated vegetable oils in cookies, crackers and deep-fried foods, may be even more harmful than saturated fat.

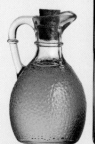
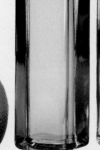

Chocolate a health food?

Studies suggest there may be health benefits to eating certain types of chocolate.

That's because chocolate contains flavonoids. These natural antioxidants — also found in tea, red wine and some fruits and vegetables — help limit the negative effects of lipoproteins, components of low-density lipoprotein (LDL or "bad") cholesterol. Flavonoids may protect your arteries and prevent heart disease and stroke.

The amount of flavonoids in chocolate depends largely on the processing. The darker the chocolate, the higher it's likely to be in flavonoids. White chocolate contains no flavonoids.

Keep in mind, though, that in addition to cocoa beans, from which chocolate is derived, most chocolate products also include ingredients such as cocoa butter, milk and sugar. These ingredients replace the amount of flavonoid in the chocolate and add fat and calories.

While chocolate may have some health benefits, it's best to keep it as an occasional snack.

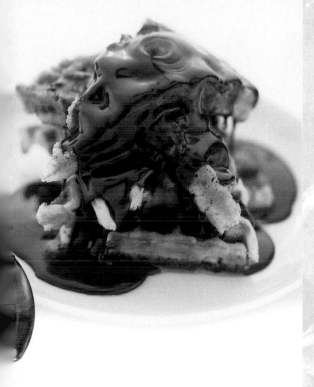

Sweets

Foods in the sweets group include candies, cakes, cookies, pies, doughnuts and other desserts. And don't forget the table sugar you add to cereal, fruit and beverages.

With sweets, small is beautiful. You won't find daily serving goals for sweets, even though they're at the pyramid's peak. That's because sweets are a high source of calories, mostly from sugar and fat, and are high in energy density, yet they offer little in terms of nutrition — they're what experts call empty calories.

You don't have to give up these foods entirely. But be smart about your selections and portion sizes. The pyramid recommends limiting sweets to 75 calories a day. Where possible, select better dessert choices, such as fig bar cookies and low-fat frozen yogurt.

Or, simply enjoy fresh fruit instead of prepared sweets or desserts. Here are some helpful calorie counts.

1 teaspoon sugar
16 calories

1 homemade oatmeal-raisin cookie
65 calories

4 ounces sorbet
95 calories

1 ounce semisweet chocolate
135 calories

Planning
for enjoyable meals

It's easy to integrate the Mayo Clinic Healthy Weight Pyramid into your daily diet and adjust it to suit your tastes. To plan menus, you just need to keep some basic principles in mind.

Know your daily calorie goal

As you plan meals for the day or the week, it's important to know approximately how many calories you should eat each day (see pages 84 and 85).

When you know your calorie goal, the daily serving recommendations for each food group will guide your menu decisions. It's also important to be familiar with serving sizes in each of the food groups. Try to include at least one serving from most food groups at each meal.

If losing weight is not one of your goals, you can still follow the principles of the Healthy Weight Pyramid to improve your health.

Plan by the week

It's more efficient to plan your meals for an entire week, especially if you shop for groceries on a weekly basis. That way, you'll know whether you have all of the ingredients on hand before you start preparing a meal.

As you plan your meals for the week, don't get hung up on hitting exact servings totals each day. It's easier to plan in terms of longer time periods. If on Monday, for example, you don't reach your fruits target, add an extra serving or two on Tuesday. You can boost your weekly greens and whole-grain totals by making some lunches and dinners vegetarian — a strategy that will also help you incorporate healthy protein sources, such as legumes and low-fat dairy products.

Make pleasure a priority

Some of your planning efforts may seem like number crunching. You're working hard to make sure that you have the right foods and the right number of servings at each meal. But don't forget that good food is one of life's pleasures. Take advantage of flavors, colors and textures to create enticing dishes. A varied selection of foods helps delight the senses.

Adapt your menus to the seasons

Whenever you can, look for recently harvested produce — asparagus, peas and cherries in the spring, peaches, sweet corn and tomatoes in midsummer, and apples, pears and beets in the fall. This way you'll promote a varied diet with the freshest foods available.

Be adventurous

Discovering new foods and flavors is part of the joy of cooking and eating, so don't be afraid to explore unfamiliar cuisines. Some of the world's most intriguing ingredients — quinoa, edamame, bok choy, bulgur — are as healthy as they are delicious. Bear in mind that the broadest range of health benefits comes from menus that feature a wide variety of nutritious foods.

Don't forget convenience foods

A healthy meal doesn't have to be complicated or time-consuming to prepare — especially if you have a busy day ahead. When meal planning, consider convenience foods for those days when there's little time to fix meals.

For example, plan at least one meal a week around a favorite convenience food, such as a frozen entree or a side dish. Just remember to be selective about which convenience foods you choose by reading the nutrition labels. Don't choose based on calories alone. Also look for items that are low in fat and that aren't loaded with sodium. Sodium is often used to help preserve food, but too much sodium isn't good for your health.

You might also find it helpful to keep on hand healthy versions of quick-cook foods such as pasta and instant brown rice.

Look for shortcuts

Another way to help simplify meal preparation and save time is to purchase pre-cut vegetables and fruits, precooked meats and packaged salads.

Frozen or canned vegetables and fruits also may come in handy for some dishes. Rinse the canned vegetables with water to help remove the sodium used in processing. To cut down on calories, buy fruit that's canned in its own juices rather than in syrup.

Be flexible

Remember that every food you eat doesn't have to be an excellent source of nutrients. Nor is it out of the question to eat high-fat, high-calorie foods on occasion. The main thing is that you choose foods that promote good health more often than those that don't.

Begin at the bottom

Vegetables and fruits should form the foundation of your diet, so you might build your daily menus on which vegetables and fruits you're planning to eat.

To make sure that you get enough fruit, aim to include at least one serving at breakfast, lunch and dinner. To make sure that you get plenty of vegetables each day, plan lunches and dinners that incorporate two or three servings each, such as a salad or a vegetable soup. Another way to pack in the vegetables is to replace some or all of the meat in casseroles or pasta dishes with vegetables.

Getting enough servings of vegetables and fruit is actually easier than it may sound, because many dishes contain more than one serving and the serving sizes are relatively small. Also keep in mind that vegetables and fruit make excellent snacks.

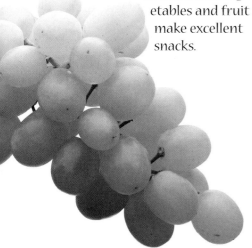

Go for the good fat

It's generally a good idea to limit the amount of fat you consume each day, especially saturated fat and trans fats. Include in your diet more healthful monosaturated fat and foods containing omega-3 fatty acids, such as fish.

To cut harmful fat and add more good fat:

- Trim visible fat from meat and remove the skin from poultry before cooking.
- Use nonstick cooking spray or nonstick cookware. When you need oil, choose olive, peanut and canola oils, or oils made from flaxseed or soybeans.
- Enhance the flavor of food without adding fat by using herbs and spices.
- Sauté vegetables in broth or wine instead of butter.
- Use vinegars on salads instead of dressings, or use low-fat or fat-free dressings.
- Substitute low-fat or fat-free dairy products for higher-fat dairy products.
- Use trans-fat-free margarine or margarine made from canola oil.
- Cook fish in paper parchment or aluminum foil to seal in flavors and juices.
- Snack on seeds and nuts

Remember those legumes

Something else to keep in mind as you do your weekly planning is to include legumes in your menus. Legumes are an impor-tant part of the protein and dairy group and are a great way to incorporate more healthy plant foods into your diet.

The term *legume* refers to a large family of plants whose seeds develop inside pods and are usually dried for ease of storage.

There are many ways that you can incorporate legumes into everyday meals. For more on legumes, see page 60.

Don't forget whole grains

Grains are the seeds of plants. When left whole, they include the endosperm, germ and bran, all of which contain beneficial nutri-ents that your body needs. Although vitamins and minerals are often added back into refined grains after the milling process, refined grains don't contain the fiber and phytochemicals that whole grains do.

Whole grains are an impor-tant part of a healthy diet because they're relatively low in fat and high in fiber. Foods high in fiber help fill you up — you eat less because your hunger is satisfied sooner.

In addition, fiber has many health benefits. It promotes healthy digestion and it may lower your risk of cardio-vascular disease, diabetes and some cancers.

When planning your menus, try to include whole-grain prod-ucts whenever you can. Some examples include oatmeal, brown rice, wild rice, whole-gain bread, whole-wheat pasta, bulgur and hulled barley.

Adapting recipes

This book provides a number of recipes to help you eat better. These recipes are a starting point toward a healthier lifestyle. As you become more comfortable with the changes in your diet, you'll likely want to experiment with new foods and recipes.

Just because you're eating healthier doesn't mean that you can't enjoy your favorite foods on occasion. You can do this by making some traditional dishes more nutritious. Chances are, you can reduce the calories and fat without greatly affecting the taste. Here are some common healthy substitutions:

If the recipe calls for	Try substituting
• Oil • Margarine • Shortening • Butter	• Low-fat vegetable broth, for frying. • For baking, replace half of the butter, margarine, shortening or oil with the same amount of apple-sauce, prune purée or commercial fat substitute. To avoid dense, soggy baked goods, don't substitute oil for butter or shortening, or diet, whipped or tub-style margarine for regular margarine.
Whole milk	1 percent or fat-free milk
Evaporated whole milk	Evaporated skim milk
Eggs	Egg substitute. A half-cup generally equals two eggs. You can use two egg whites for each whole egg in most recipes, too.
Sour cream	Fat-free plain yogurt or low-fat sour cream. Fat-free sour cream isn't intended for baking.
Cream cheese	Light cream cheese, Neufchatel cheese or low-fat cottage cheese puréed until smooth. Fat-free cream cheese isn't intended for baking.
Chocolate	Cocoa and oil or corn syrup. Instead of one square of unsweetened chocolate, use 3 tablespoons of cocoa and 1 tablespoon corn syrup. Instead of one square of semisweet chocolate, use 3 tablespoons of cocoa and 1 tablespoon. oil. Or use less chocolate and break it into smaller pieces for greater dispersal.
Sugar	In most baked goods you can reduce the amount of sugar by one-half without affecting the food's texture or taste. Because sugar increases moisture in baked goods, make sure you use no less than 1/4 cup of sugar, honey or molasses for every cup of flour.
Flour	Whole-grain flour. It can be substituted for regular flour in many recipes, such as bread or muffins. Whole-grain flour is higher in fiber than is regular flour.

Understanding nutrition labels

The Nutrition Facts food label is a great tool to help you seek out foods that are healthy. At first glance, the numbers and percentages on the label may look intimidating. But as you become more familiar with its format, you'll find that the label informs you about the contents of a product and helps you compare the nutritional qualities of similar products.

Serving size. Serving size information is based on the amount of this particular food people typically eat. Serving sizes are based on standard household measurements, such as cups, ounces and pieces. Similar foods usually have similar serving sizes.

Calories. The calories listed relate to one serving of this particular food. In this example, there are 130 calories in six wafers. It's important to be mindful of calorie options when comparing like products. This label also reveals how many calories in one serving come from fat. In this example, 40 of the 130 calories come from fat.

Nutrients. Food companies must list, at the minimum, the amounts and types of fat, total fat, saturated fat, cholesterol, sodium, total carbohydrate, dietary fiber, sugars, protein, vitamins A and C, calcium and iron that are contained in one serving of a product. Too much or too little of these nutrients can have an impact on your health.

- Limit these nutrients: total fat, saturated fat, trans fat, cholesterol and sodium.

- Get plenty of these nutrients: dietary fiber, vitamin A, vitamin C, calcium and iron.

Percent Daily Value. The Daily Value numbers (%DV) on a Nutrition Facts label tell you how much of the daily recommended amounts of nutrients are contained in one serving of this food. These percentages are based on a 2,000-calories-a-day diet. For example, the label pictured here indicates that the 4.5 grams of total fat in one serving is 7 percent of all fat that an average person should consume in a day. That means there's 93 percent remaining total fat for the day. You may consume more or less than 2,000 calories a day, but you can still use the %DV as a frame of reference.

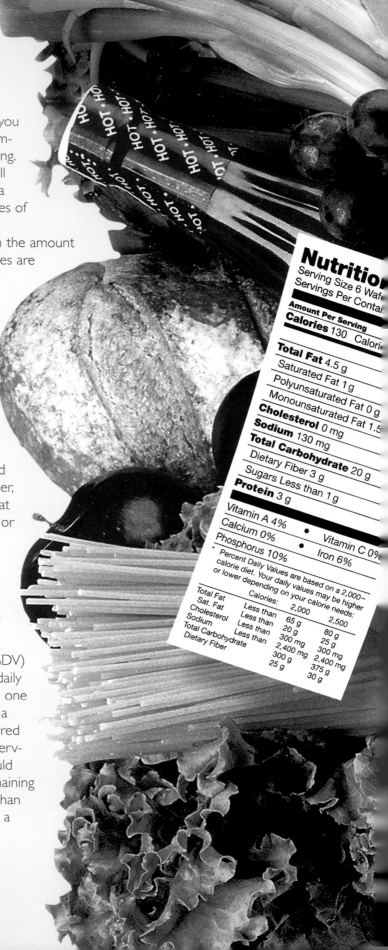

Label lingo

It can be confusing when you see terms such as *reduced fat* and *low fat* on food labels because no definition or explanation is provided. Is reduced fat the same as low fat? Not necessarily. Be sure to check the nutrition label.

The Food and Drug Administration (FDA) defines and regulates the use of terms involving nutrient content. Manufacturers can use these terms to draw your attention to foods that are high or low in various nutrients. Here's what some common terms mean:

Food label claim	What it means	Related terms	Specific examples
Free	Product is absolutely free of the nutrient in question, or if the nutrient is in the food, the amount must be insignificant.	• Without • Negligible source of • Dietarily insignificant source of • No, zero, non	• Fat-free: 0.5 grams (g) or less • Cholesterol-free: 2 milligrams (mg) or less • Sodium-free: 5 mg or less • Sugar-free: 0.5 g or less
Light	• Must have half the fat or one-third fewer calories than the regular product. • Must have at least 50 percent less sodium than the regular product and be low in calories and fat.	• Lite	• Light sour cream • Light in sodium
Low	Meets the definition of "low" if food can be eaten frequently without exceeding dietary guidelines for fat, saturated fat, cholesterol, sodium or calories.	• Little • Few • Contains a small amount of • Low source of	• Low fat: 3 g or less • Low in saturated fat: 1 g or less • Low in sodium: 140 mg or less • Very low sodium: 35 mg or less • Low calorie: 40 calories or less • Low cholesterol: 20 mg or less and 2 g or less of saturated fat
Reduced	Food must contain at least 25 percent less of a nutrient or calories than the regular product. Beware, the regular product may be very high in sodium, fat and calories.	• Less • Fewer	• Reduced sodium • Reduced fat • Fewer calories

Adapted from the Food and Drug Administration, Food Labeling Guide, 1999

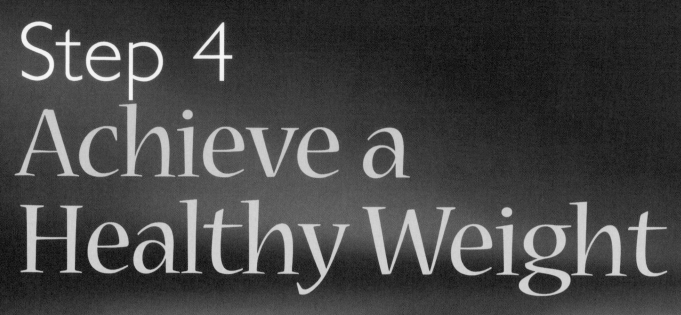

Step 4
Achieve a Healthy Weight

A visit with Dr. Donald Hensrud

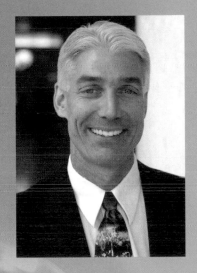

Donald Hensrud, M.D.
Preventive Medicine

That there are so many diet plans available attests to the fact that few of them work for most people or are effective over the long term. The term *diet* often implies something that's restrictive, negative and, therefore, temporary. Many diets will help people lose weight over a short period of time, but usually the weight is regained and there's no improvement in health.

Diets may work in different ways — some restrict fat or carbohydrates, some restrict the amount of food you eat, and others restrict certain foods, such as fruit after lunch. Regardless of the specific recommendations, what eventually happens is that people go off their diet. Perhaps this is because of boredom or lack of motivation or, more likely, because the diet is too restrictive and doesn't offer any variety (How much cabbage soup can one person eat?).

If you really want to lose weight and keep it off, the best approach is to focus on lifestyle changes and develop an eating plan that's enjoyable, yet healthy and low in calories. This approach will result in weight loss that you can live with — that is, that you can maintain over a long period of time.

Achieving a healthy weight takes work — or more correctly, planning — but the rewards are great. Over time, your efforts will turn into a sustainable, healthy lifestyle that can improve your nutrition and level of physical activity. You'll feel better immediately and reduce your health risks. More importantly, this change in lifestyle should and can be an enjoyable way for you to live.

Q: Is calorie counting still the best way to lose weight?

A: Calories do count, but virtually everyone underestimates how many calories he or she consumes each day. And people trying to lose weight may underestimate their calorie intake even more. In addition, some people become so focused on calories they lose sight of the big picture — adopting a more healthy lifestyle. If counting calories works for you, use that approach. If you're not a calorie counter, there are other methods you can use, such as keeping track of food servings, as we discuss in the following pages. By eating the recommended number of servings from each food group, the same objective can be accomplished — weight loss from eating fewer calories.

Q: Is being 'a little overweight' really harmful to your health?

A: In science, studies often don't produce the same results. While a couple of studies indicate that being a little overweight may not be harmful, the vast majority of the evidence points to overweight and obesity as having adverse health effects, including how long you'll live and your quality of life. There are many complications from overweight or obesity that impact people's quality of life and that don't show up in the mortality statistics — such as degenerative arthritis in even moderately overweight people, which can decrease mobility. It's true that the greater the weight, the greater the adverse health effects. So, someone who's mildly overweight isn't at the same health risks as someone who's markedly obese. However, once people become mildly overweight, it can be difficult to stay there and they may be on their way to obesity.

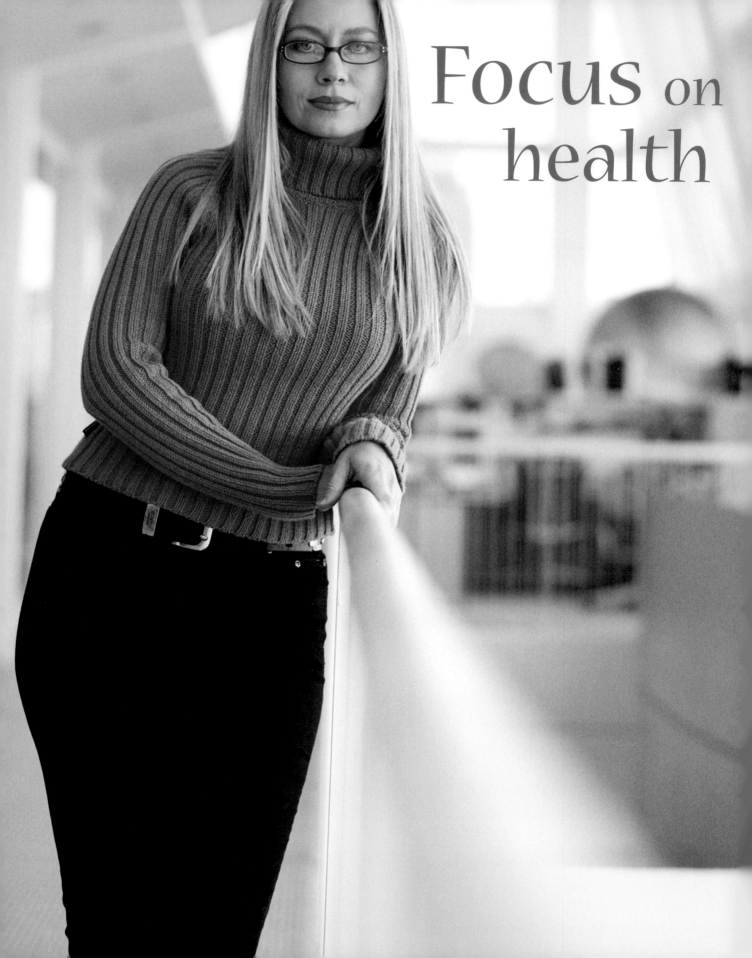

Focus on health

When it comes to weight loss, there's no shortage of advice. Cruise through any bookstore or browse through any magazine rack, and you're bound to come across the latest and greatest cure for being overweight. Some even work — for a while.

But for a moment, put aside thoughts of dieting and looking thinner, and think about what it means to simply be healthy.

Most diets focus only on what you eat — labeling some foods as good and others as bad. The main goal is to lose pounds. Unfortunately, as you likely know from personal experience, those lost pounds usually come back.

Mayo Clinic has developed a common-sense approach to weight control, based on the knowledge and expertise of its clinicians, that encourages smart decisions and healthy behaviors grounded on fundamentals of the Mayo Clinic Healthy Weight Pyramid. It's not a diet that you end up going on and off. It's a lifestyle program to better health that you'll enjoy for a lifetime.

The following pages will show you how to get started. The first section in this step helps you determine a healthy weight. The next part shows you how to control calories through a balanced diet, moderate food portions and daily physical activity. The Mayo Clinic Healthy Weight Pyramid, an essential part of your plan, is discussed on pages 52-63 in Step 3 of this book. A third section includes guidelines for staying motivated and changing behaviors that can impede your progress or throw you completely off the program. Finally, in the last section, you'll find practical, easy-to-prepare menus that you can adapt to your personal tastes.

The Mayo Clinic approach recognizes that successful, long-term weight loss needs to focus on more than the food you eat and the pounds you lose. It needs to focus on your health.

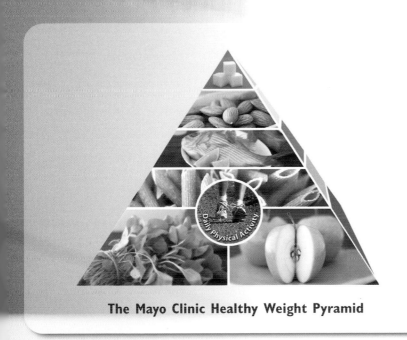

The Mayo Clinic Healthy Weight Pyramid

Is my weight healthy?

A common question for many people is, "How do I know if I'm at a healthy weight — a weight that's right for me?"

Technically, a healthy weight means that you have the right amount of body fat in relation to your overall body mass. Body mass includes bone, muscle, fluid and fat. Health experts consider the right amount of fat for adult women to be about 20 percent of their total body mass, and for adult men, around 13 percent to 17 percent.

Practically, a healthy weight means a weight that reduces your risk of disease and allows you to look and feel good.

Stepping on the scale will tell you your total weight, but not how much of your weight is fat. The scale also doesn't tell you where you're carrying most of that fat, such as around your abdomen or your buttocks.

In determining your health risks and whether you're at a healthy weight, two factors that are equally important to your total weight, if not more so, are the percentage of your weight that's fat and the location of that fat.

So how do you know if you have too much body fat? The most accurate method for determining body fat percentage is to have a body fat analysis, which can be complicated and is often expensive. Although less certain, a more common approach for estimating body fat takes into consideration three key factors:

- Your body mass index
- The circumference of your waist
- Your personal medical history

Body mass index

Body mass index (BMI) is a tool for indicating if your weight is healthy or unhealthy.

The mathematical calculation used to determine BMI takes into account both your weight and your height. Your BMI is formulated by dividing your weight by your height squared.

Although BMI doesn't distinguish between fat and muscle, it more closely reflects measures of body fat than does total weight alone.

You may already know your BMI number from having taken the health assessment in Step 1. If you haven't taken the assessment, turn now to page 13 to determine your body mass index. According to the table shown, are you:

- Underweight
- At a healthy weight
- Overweight
- Obese

For most people, their body mass index provides a fairly accurate approximation of their body composition, but it's not always a good match. Some people may have a high BMI but relatively little body fat. For example, many athletes have high BMIs that appear to classify them as being overweight, or even obese. This is because vigorous athletic training has turned most of their weight into lean muscle mass.

By the same token, there may be some people who have a BMI in the "healthy" range but who carry a high percentage of body fat, which places them at higher risk of health conditions.

Your weight and your health

The more excess fat you carry, the greater your risk of developing certain health conditions. Among these conditions are:

High blood pressure. Obese individuals are twice as likely to develop high blood pressure (hypertension) as are individuals who maintain a healthy weight.

Abnormal blood fats. Being overweight is associated with low levels of high-density lipoprotein (HDL, or "good") cholesterol and high levels of triglycerides (another type of fat) in your bloodstream.

Type 2 diabetes. More than 80 percent of adults with type 2 diabetes are overweight or obese.

Cardiovascular disease. A weight gain of just 10 to 20 pounds can increase your risk of heart and blood vessel problems by 25 percent. A gain of 45 pounds or more increases the risk by more than 250 percent.

Other complications. If you're overweight, your health is at increased risk of other conditions, including osteoarthritis, gallstones and sleep apnea. Most types of cancer are associated with being overweight. In women, these especially include cancers of the breast, uterus, colon and gallbladder.

It's all about location

For years, scientists have sought to understand why an apple shape — that is, extra fat carried around the waist — places someone at a higher risk of many weight-related conditions. The prevailing theory was that excess fat surrounding the abdominal organs flooded the bloodstream with increased levels of fatty acids, leading to a host of problems.

Studies directed by Michael Jensen, M.D., head of Mayo Clinic's Endocrine Research Unit, have refocused that theory. Dr. Jensen's work suggests that subcutaneous fat — the fat that's stored directly under the skin in the upper body — can be a greater source of fat in the bloodstream.

With this big picture in hand, scientists are digging deeper with studies that are focused at the cellular and molecular level. It is hoped these findings will help researchers better understand the mechanisms that regulate fat storage and perhaps even discover ways to remove excess fat.

Other research being conducted by Dr. Jensen tracks the pathways of fat molecules as they travel from the bloodstream into the internal structures of a cell, as well as the effects of overeating on fat distribution.

Waist measurement

Medical conditions associated with obesity include high blood pressure, high cholesterol, coronary artery disease, stroke, diabetes and certain types of cancer. You're at a higher risk of these conditions not only because of the amount of fat you carry but also by the location of that fat on your body.

Your body has a nearly unlimited capacity to store fat, and that excess fat often shows up in your midsection. Fat distribution can be described in terms of an apple shape or pear shape. If you carry most of your fat around your waist or upper body, you're referred to as apple shaped. If you carry most of your fat around your hips and thighs or lower body, you're referred to as pear shaped.

In general, when it comes to your health, it's better to have a pear shape than an apple shape. Having an apple shape means your abdominal fat is out of proportion with your total body fat. When you carry more fat in and around your abdominal organs, you increase your risk of disease, even if your BMI falls within a normal range. If you have a pear shape, your risks of these conditions aren't as high.

To determine whether you're carrying too much weight around your middle, you'll need to measure your waist. Find the highest point on each hipbone and measure around your abdomen just above those points.

A measurement exceeding 40 inches (102 centimeters) in men or 35 inches (88 centimeters) in women indicates an apple shape and increased health risks. Your risk is even greater if you have a BMI of 25 or higher. The table on page 76 can help you determine whether your waistline is a concern.

Although these cutoffs of 40 and 35 inches are useful guides, there's nothing magical about them. It's enough to know that the bigger the waistline, the greater your health risks.

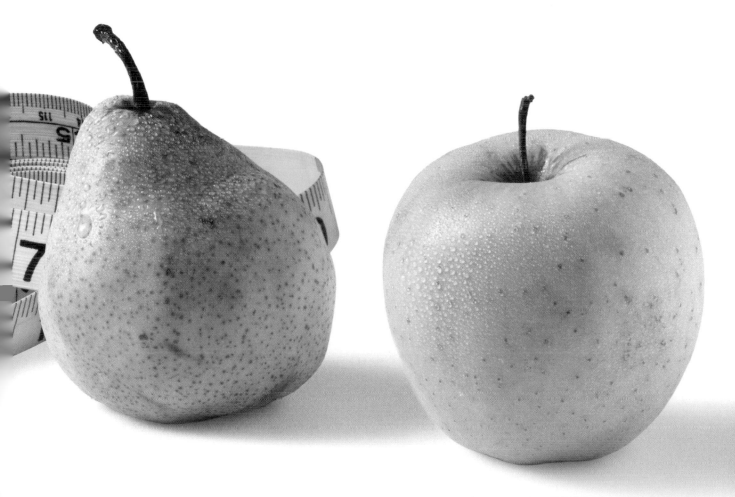

Medical history

An evaluation of your personal medical history is also important for getting a complete picture of your weight status. Information from your medical history can help your doctor assess your risk of weight-related conditions.

This evaluation takes place between you and your doctor. Some questions that your doctor may ask include:

- Do you have a health condition, such as high blood pressure or diabetes, that would improve if you lost weight?
- Do you have a family history of obesity, cardiovascular disease, diabetes, high blood pressure or sleep apnea? A yes response could mean that you may be at increased risk of a particular disease.
- Have you gained a lot of weight since high school? Even people with normal BMIs may be at increased risk of weight-related conditions if they've gained more than 10 pounds since they were young adults.
- Do you smoke cigarettes or are you physically inactive? Either of these risk factors — smoking or inactivity (being sedentary) — may compound health risks associated with excess weight.

Think of your BMI number and your waist measurement as snapshots of your current health. A medical history completes the picture by revealing your long-term risk of weight-related diseases.

A healthy weight for you

If your BMI shows that you're not overweight (a BMI number under 25), if you're not carrying too much weight around your abdomen, and if you answered no to all of the medical history questions, there's probably little advantage to changing your weight. It's probably healthy right now.

If your BMI is between 25 and 29 or your waist circumference exceeds the healthy guidelines, you'll probably benefit from losing some weight, especially if you answered yes to one of the medical history questions.

If your BMI is 30 or more, you're considered obese. This puts you at high risk of weight-related conditions. Losing weight will improve your health and reduce your risk of these illnesses.

Your BMI	Your waist measurements			
	Women		*Men*	
	35 inches or less	Exceeding 35 inches	40 inches or less	Exceeding 40 inches
25 to 29.9	Increased	High	Increased	High
30 to 34.9	High	Very high	High	Very high
35 to 39.9	Very high	Very high	Very high	Very high
40 or higher	Extremely high	Extremely high	Extremely high	Extremely high

If your BMI is between 18.5 and 24.9, your health is likely not at risk from your weight. A BMI of 25 and over may put you at risk of serious health problems. Note: Asians with a BMI of 23 or higher may have an increased risk of health problems.

Accepting your healthy weight

When it comes to weight and body image, you may be tougher on yourself than anyone else is. You may be preoccupied with losing a few more pounds — even if you never actually do anything about it. You may focus on physical features that you don't like. You dwell on the imperfections, the wrinkles, the extra weight — and not all the positive attributes.

You prefer instead to imagine having a perfect body with a thin waist, toned legs and washboard abs   a body you'll be proud to take to the beach. Sounds good, doesn't it? A perfect vision. And that's exactly what it is — a vision — because a perfect body is nearly impossible to attain.

Most of us aren't supermodels or professional bodybuilders. We're real people with real bodies — complex in their wonders and flaws. Unfortunately, it's the gulf between the ideal and reality that causes so much dissatisfaction and discouragement.

What if the weight category indicated by a BMI number is not quite what you had envisioned for yourself? There's a saying that goes, "Happiness comes not from what you have, but from how you regard what you have." The path to a healthy weight starts by accepting that every body is different, strongly influenced by genetics and environment. Even if everyone ate the same food and did the same exercises for a lifetime, people's bodies would still come in all shapes and sizes.

You can also focus on what makes you feel good about your body. If you're eating balanced meals, getting exercise and have the energy to do the things you want to do, you're already on the right track. Trust that, by staying focused on your health, the pounds will take care of themselves and you'll achieve a weight that's right for you.

You can learn to break a negative mind-set with the following suggestions:

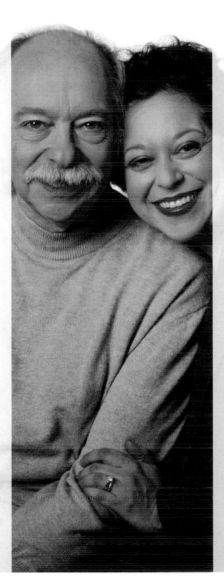

- Don't let your perceptions dictate how you live your life. Realize it's your own discomfort stopping you, not what others are thinking.

- Play up the positives. There's a lot to like about you. Remind yourself that there's more to you than clothing size.

- Think of a skill, talent or personality trait that you take special pride in. Then fill in the blank: "I like the fact that I have (or can do) _____."

- Give yourself a break. Hop off the scale and stop bad-mouthing yourself. Appreciate what you see in the mirror and avoid negative "double takes" of yourself.

- Accept compliments. Don't push away kind words and practice saying thank you

- Wear what you like. Don't worry about what's appropriate for your age, status or body type.

- Pick friends wisely. Associate with people who accept you as you are.

- Give yourself time. You didn't develop a negative body image overnight. Don't expect an instant about-face.

- Listen to your doctor, who can help you — either directly or through referral to a dietitian or nutrition specialist — to determine a weight that best suits your body type and enhances your long-term health.

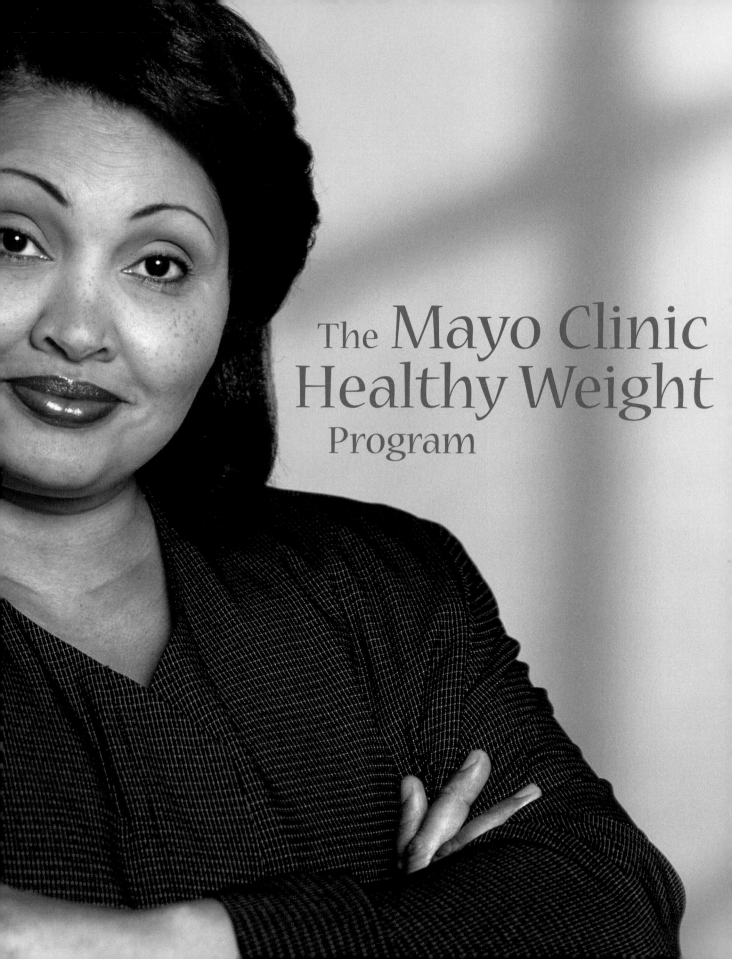

The **Mayo Clinic**
Healthy Weight
Program

So you've decided that it's time to lose weight. Maybe it's because your doctor has advised you to lose a few pounds. Maybe you've looked in the mirror and you don't like what you see. Perhaps you simply want to weigh the same as you did when you were in college.

There are tons of reasons why people want to lose weight. The problem is knowing how to do it.

The Mayo Clinic Healthy Weight Program is a practical guide to weight control. It requires your commitment and a willingness to make lifestyle changes. But it's a program that you can enjoy.

To get started, you'll need to follow these five steps:

1.) Assess your readiness
2.) Establish a weight goal
3.) Identify a daily calorie goal
4.) Calculate your daily food servings
5.) Assess your fitness level

Seem like a lot of work just to get started? Actually, each step takes only a few minutes.

Assess your readiness

Motivation is an emotional incentive to take action. It pushes you to put the familiar diet dictums of "eat less" and "exercise more" into practice.

Your chance of success is greater if your motivations are based on what you want for yourself and not on what others expect of you. The assessment on the following page can help gauge your motivation.

Once you're ready, here are some strategies to help bolster and sustain your motivation:

- **Emphasize the positives.** Focus on the good things about losing weight — such as more energy and improved health — and not on what you consider the negatives.
- **Prioritize.** Don't set yourself up for failure by trying to lose weight while distracted by other concerns. Resolve those other problems first.
- **Focus on small steps.** Set realistic, attainable goals that you can achieve and feel good about. When you meet your goals, give yourself a small reward. Once you've achieved a goal, set a new, more challenging one.
- **Steer clear of dietary gimmicks.** Over-the-counter pills and special food combinations aren't the answer to long-term weight control. You want to incorporate healthy behaviors into your lifestyle, not rely on gimmicks.
- **Seek out support.** Don't feel you have to go it alone. Exercising with a friend or family member can help keep you motivated.
- **Remind yourself you're not looking for a quick fix.** Healthy weight loss is slow and steady weight loss that occurs over time. Remind yourself that quick weight loss is usually followed by quick weight regain a short time later.

Slow and steady wins the race

Weight loss is best when it's gradual. Think in terms of losing no more than 1 to 2 pounds a week. That's a goal that's realistic, achievable and less stressful on you physically and emotionally. A loss of just 5 percent to 10 percent of your body weight — no matter what your weight — brings important benefits to your health and improves your quality of life.

Here's a practical perspective on weight loss: Because 3,500 calories equals about 1 pound of body fat, you need to burn 3,500 calories more than you consume in a week in order to lose 1 pound. That calculates to about 500 fewer calories a day. Conversely, when you eat 3,500 excess calories, you gain 1 pound.

You've undoubtedly heard statistics about how only a few people succeed at losing weight and keeping it off. Don't let that discourage you. Sure, you're taking on a tough challenge — possibly one of the hardest you'll ever tackle. But with a little knowledge, a positive attitude and a good plan, you can do it. The pounds will take care of themselves. Even if you don't reach your "ideal" weight, you'll be much healthier than you were before.

Are you ready to lose weight?

Starting a weight program before you're sure that you're ready can set you up for failure. To the contrary, you don't want to put off your start date any longer than necessary. The following questions may help you make this decision.

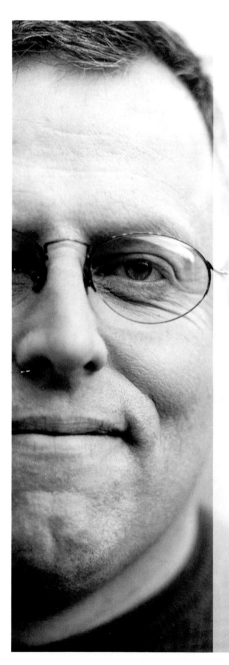

1. How motivated are you to lose weight?
   a. Extremely motivated
   b. Quite motivated
   c. Somewhat motivated
   d. Slightly motivated

2. Considering the amount of stress affecting your life right now, to what extent can you focus on weight loss and on making lifestyle changes?
   a. Can focus easily
   b. Can focus well
   c. Uncertain
   d. Can focus somewhat

3. Weight loss is recommended at a rate of 1 to 2 pounds a week. How realistic do you think your expectations are about how much weight you would like to lose and how quickly you want to lose it?
   a. Very realistic
   b. Moderately realistic
   c. Somewhat realistic
   d. Somewhat or very unrealistic

4. Aside from holiday feasts, have you ever eaten a large amount of food rapidly and felt afterward that this eating was out of control?
   a. No
   b. Yes

5. If you answered yes to the question above, how often have you eaten like this during the last year?
   a. About once a month or less
   b. A few times a month
   c. About once a week
   d. About three times a week or more

6. Do you eat for emotional reasons, for example, when you feel anxious, depressed, angry or lonely? Do you celebrate good feelings by overeating?
   a. Never or rarely
   b. Occasionally
   c. Frequently
   d. Always

7. How confident are you that you can make changes in your eating habits and sustain them?
   a. Completely confident
   b. Highly confident
   c. Somewhat confident
   d. Slightly confident

8. How confident are you that you can exercise regularly?
   a. Completely confident
   b. Highly confident
   c. Somewhat confident
   d. Slightly confident

Evaluating your readiness to lose weight

- If most of your responses are a and b, you're probably ready to start losing weight.

- If most of your responses are b and c, consider if you're ready to start a weight-loss program or if you should wait for a better time.

- If most of your responses are d, you may want to hold off on your start date. Reassess your readiness again in a short while.

- If your answer to question 5 was b, c or d, you may want to discuss this with your doctor.

Other eating plans

Americans spend billions of dollars each year on diet products and services, ranging from low-calorie soft drinks to fat-free foods to diet books, all in search of a magic bullet that helps them shed pounds.

Most people who diet find it's a never-ending roller coaster ride. At first, it seems easy enough to lose weight quickly with most popular diets, often because they restrict your total calorie intake. A calorie is a calorie, no matter where it comes from or how it's consumed, and when you eat fewer calories than your body regularly burns, you're bound to lose some weight.

Unfortunately, people often find diets hard to sustain for long periods of time, in part because they tire of avoiding certain foods, loading up on others or feeling deprived and hungry. And their diet is often temporary, something to follow for a certain amount of time before returning to former ways. As a result, the lost pounds come right back once the diet stops.

Some of the popular diets in circulation today include:

Low-fat diets

Cutting down on high-fat foods can help reduce your daily calories and thus help you lose weight. So why don't these plans always work? Even a low-fat diet can lead to weight gain when people ignore the total amount of calories they're eating and regularly exceed their daily calorie goals. Too many calories from any source, low-fat foods included, can add pounds.

Low-carb diets

Followers of these eating plans believe that a decrease in dietary carbs results in lower insulin levels, which causes the body to burn stored fat tissue for energy.

Many people, in fact, do lose weight on low-carb diets, but the weight loss probably isn't related to blood sugar levels. More likely, it's related to three factors:

- **Loss of water weight.** When your body burns the stored fat tissue, much of the initial weight loss is due to the release of water in glycogen — a loss that usually lasts only a few days.

- **Decreased appetite.** Burning fat without carbohydrates creates a buildup of byproducts in your bloodstream (ketosis). In a state of ketosis, your appetite may decrease. Also, fat increases your sense of being full.

- **Reduced calories.** Most low-carb diets reduce your calorie intake because they limit carbohydrate-containing foods.

Well known low-carb diets include the Atkins diet, Zone diet and Protein Power.

Glycemic-index diets

The glycemic index ranks carbohydrate-containing foods based on their effects on blood sugar. Similar to the theory behind low-carb diets, most glycemic-index diets claim that lowering blood sugar levels leads to weight loss.

You may have difficulty following a diet that emphasizes only foods with a low glycemic-index ranking. Many factors other than food influence your blood sugar level, including your age and weight, the type of food preparation and the portion size.

A well known glycemic-index diet is the South Beach diet.

Meal providers

Some people have a difficult time knowing what they're supposed to eat. Busy schedules leave little time for meal preparation. In such cases, relying on ready-made meals eaten at home may deserve consideration. These providers include Jenny Craig and NutriSystem.

Meal replacements

Plans such as Slim-Fast call for you to eat one sensible meal each day and replace other meals with products such as their meal replacement shakes. Following this type of program can lead to long-term weight loss.

Group approaches

You don't have to lose weight alone. Group programs such as Weight Watchers can support your efforts, giving you eating plans, exercise recommendations and support from others on the same dietary path.

The Mayo Clinic Healthy Weight Program is focused mainly on lifestyle. What you eat is certainly a big part of this approach. But it's also about permanently changing behaviors from unhealthy to healthy ones.

Establish a weight goal

So, how much weight would you like to lose? Perhaps it's 10 to 20 pounds. Or maybe your goal is more ambitious — you'd like to lose 50 or even 100 pounds.

Goal setting is a way to meet these expectations. But your expectations must be realistic, and include some goals that are achievable within a short period of time. Goals that are unrealistic or too long-term just disappoint you when you don't meet them.

For many overweight people, a reasonable goal is to lose about 10 percent of their starting body weight. Permanent behavior change can help meet this goal. And many people experience noticeable improvements in their health with that amount of weight loss.

Always be willing to reassess and adjust goals, whether you progress or struggle with your program. You will lose the weight. Your life will change. But it takes time.

Weighing in

Too many people think that pounds lost is the only way to judge their progress in a weight program. That's why weighing in is often such an emotional experience. If you find that you've gained weight, you may feel depressed and ultimately quit trying. If your weight stays the same, you may become disillusioned or bored.

Success isn't measured just by the bathroom scale. Consider the fact that, even with minor weight loss, you're healthier. You have more energy, and you feel better about yourself. These are wonderful benefits in addition to weight loss.

How regularly should you weigh yourself? That depends. Checking the scale too often can cause people to obsess about daily weight fluctuations. Not checking enough may indicate a lack of commitment. A common rule of thumb is to weigh yourself once a week.

However, if you feel that you should weigh in more often — a couple of times a week or even daily — that's OK. Just remember that it's the general trend of your weight that's important, not the day-to-day fluctuations.

To help get an accurate account of your weight, be consistent as to when you weigh in from week to week. Choose a convenient day and time and stick to that schedule. Record the number of pounds lost or gained on a copy of the weight record, shown on the opposite page. If it's helpful, include comments on your record. For example, you might indicate when you started exercising more, or when you were traveling or on vacation — not following your daily routine.

You'll weigh yourself twice in the first week of the program: on your start date and later at the end of the week. Your weight on the start date is the only number you'll need to remember — write it down and mark it as "0" on the weight record.

Occasionally, take time to review your progress. If you find that you're not meeting your weight goals, don't be too hard on yourself. Try to identify situations or factors that may be working against you and see what you can do to avoid or prevent their recurrence.

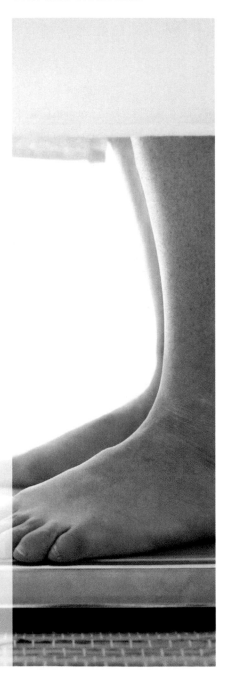

Weight record

Date →

Starting weight: —————

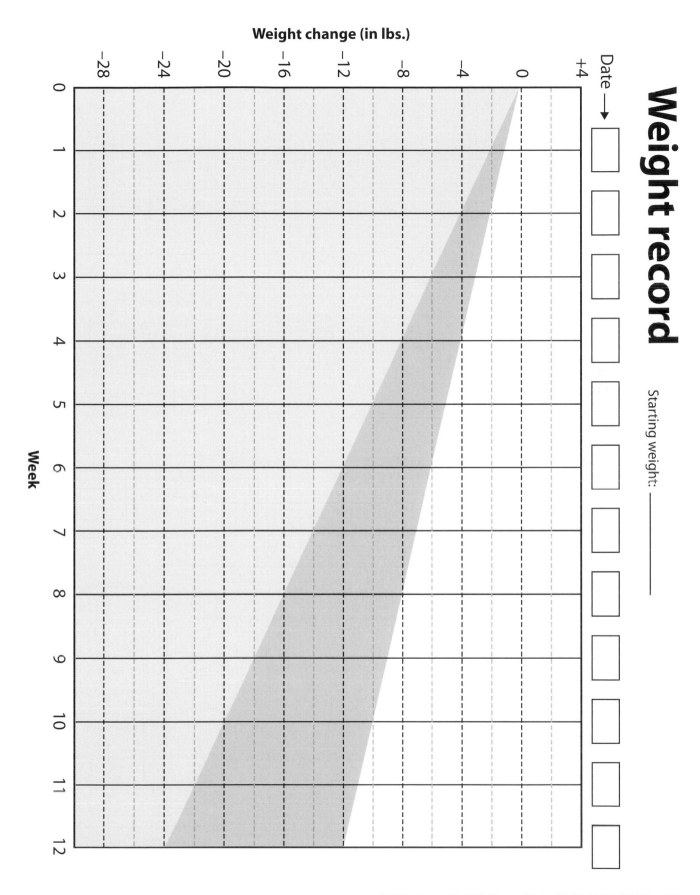

Weight change (in lbs.)

+4
0
-4
-8
-12
-16
-20
-24
-28

Week

0 1 2 3 4 5 6 7 8 9 10 11 12

Identify a calorie goal

The number of calories you regularly eat are reflected in the week-to-week changes of your weight record. Extra calories, obviously, can turn into extra pounds. So, it's important to regulate how many calories you eat each day in order to lose or maintain weight. If you can regularly meet these daily calorie goals, you should be able to reach your overall weight goal.

Theoretically, if the calories you eat are the same amount as the calories your body burns each day, you'll maintain your weight. For most people, this ranges from about 1,600 to 2,400 calories daily. The table below indicates, on average, the daily calorie goals for individuals seeking to maintain their weight.

What if you plan to lose weight? If you could eat 500 fewer calories than you generally consume each day, you could lose about a pound a week. That's because 3,500 calories (500 calories x 7 days) equals 1 pound of body fat. Losing 1 to 2 pounds a week is considered a healthy rate of weight loss.

But this method requires too much calculation. Here's a simpler approach: An average woman who wants to lose weight should set her daily calorie goal at 1,200 calories. An average man should set his daily calorie goal at 1,400 calories.

These calorie goals are good starting points for most people who weigh 250 pounds or less when they begin their weight programs. The calorie levels can be adjusted, based on your health risks and on how quickly you want to lose weight.

Weight loss at this rate puts less stress on your body than does a more drastic reduction in calories. If you feel exceptionally hungry, or you lose weight too quickly, you may consider jumping up to the next higher calorie level, as indicated by the table on page 85.

If you weigh more than 250 pounds, you'll need a slightly higher calorie goal. Refer to the table on the next page for the recommended daily calorie level to help you lose weight.

Daily calorie goals under 1,200 for women and 1,400 for men generally aren't recommended. If your daily calorie intake is too low, you may not be getting enough of the nutrients you need for good health. It's tempting to starve yourself to lose weight quickly, but doing so is not a healthy or effective long-term strategy.

Daily calorie goals for maintaining weight

On average, daily calorie goals for people seeking to maintain their weight are as follows:

Calories	
1,600	Children ages 2 to 6, most women and some older adults
2,000	Average adult
2,200	Older children, teenage girls, active women and most men
2,400	Teenage boys and active men

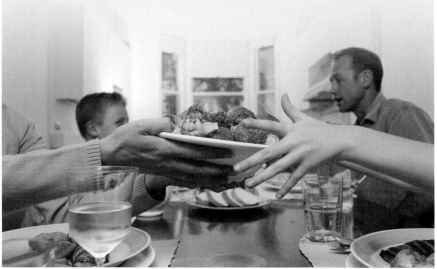

Adjusting your daily calorie goal

The recommendations of the Healthy Weight Pyramid can assist everyone's situation. They aren't part of a rigid program that people must conform to. Rather, the pyramid is a flexible tool that can personalize a weight program and guide your food choices. It can assist people with different physical characteristics, activity levels, lifestyle needs, health risks and calorie goals to eat healthier.

Over time, people's calorie goals will change. In other words, tools such as the food pyramid and the calorie goal tables provide structure to your weight program, but you should be prepared to adjust these guidelines. Daily calorie goals can be adjusted to higher levels if you become too hungry during the day or if you've reached your target weight and your goal now is to maintain that weight.

Keep in mind that you can slightly adjust the daily servings, depending on whether you're meeting your weight goals and on how full you feel. For example, there's no limit on the number of servings you can eat from the vegetables group and the fruits group (with the exception of fruit juice and dried fruits).

And rather than restricting sweets consumption to only a small amount each day, you can eat a dessert on one day and then skip sweets entirely for several following days.

Of course, your servings totals may also be affected by how active you are from day to day. An afternoon of strenuous exercise obviously burns more calories than does the same amount of time spent sitting in an office chair. Use good discretion and don't get too hung up on the daily totals.

If you eventually reach a point where you find that you're not losing weight anymore even though your diet and exercise routines haven't changed, you may have lost all of the weight that you will lose at your current calorie level. Sticking with your current plan will help you maintain your weight, but not cause you to lose more.

If you still want to lose more weight, reduce your daily calorie level by 200 calories, providing this doesn't put you below 1,200 calories. And gradually increase the amount of time you exercise daily by 15 to 30 minutes.

Daily calorie levels for healthy weight loss

	Weight in pounds	Starting calorie level			
		1,200	1,400	1,600	1,800
Women	250 or less	X			
	251 to 300		X		
	301 or more			X	
Men	250 or less		X		
	251 to 300			X	
	301 or more				X

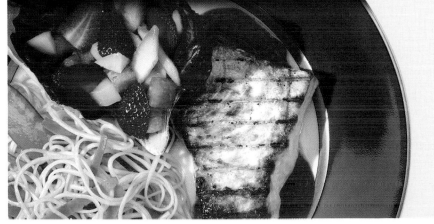

Calculate daily food servings

In learning about diet and nutrition, you're sure to come across the term *serving*. A serving isn't the amount of food you choose to eat or the amount that's put on your plate. This is called a portion. A serving is a specific amount of food, defined by standard measurements such as cups, ounces or pieces — for example, medium or small pieces of fruit. Average serving sizes for the different food groups are shown on the opposite page.

Your ability to monitor the number of servings you eat at meals is key to meeting your daily calorie goal. Due to the variation in calorie content, serving sizes vary from one food group to the next. For example, an average serving of vegetables is about 1 cup and an average serving of carbohydrates is about ½ cup.

You also need to be aware that the measurements vary within a single food group. For example, ½ cup of baby carrots, 1 cup of broccoli, and 2 cups of shredded lettuce are all equivalent to one vegetable serving. An extended list of the serving sizes for different food groups can be found on pages 119-123.

Keeping all the food groups and measurements straight may seem overwhelming. Don't panic! Serving sizes aren't as complex as they may seem. You don't need to have the entire list memorized in your head. Start with the foods you use most frequently. You'll be surprised at how quickly you'll retain this knowledge and be able to expand your serving list. But it takes some practice.

Very often, a portion of food will contain several servings of different food groups. For example, a portion of chicken casserole may contain various servings of vegetables, protein and dairy, carbohydrates and fats.

Your best estimate of the different serving sizes is usually sufficient. You may be able to refer to a recipe or ingredients list on the package. Be on the lookout for what are known as hidden calories — the extra calories from ingredients you may not be aware of in sauces, spreads, gravies and condiments.

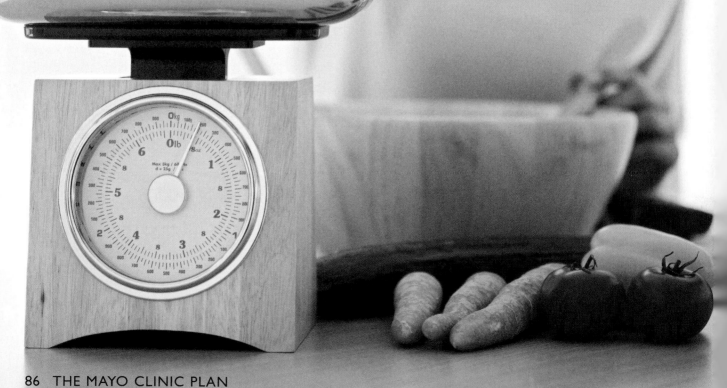

Introduction to serving sizes

An important part of eating healthy is understanding how much of a particular food makes up a serving. Many people envision servings to be larger than they are, and they eat more than they should. This page provides some visual cues to help you gauge serving sizes. On pages 119-123 you'll find a list of serving sizes for a number of foods. Use these serving lists to help you develop daily menus. Or, if you're following the menus in this book and you don't care for some of the foods on the menu, use the lists to substitute a food item for another item within the same food group.

Vegetables	Visual cue
• 1 cup broccoli	1 baseball
• 2 cups raw, leafy greens	2 baseballs

Fruits	Visual cue
• 1/2 cup sliced fruit	Tennis ball
• 1 small apple or medium orange	

Carbohydrates	Visual cue
• 1/2 cup pasta, rice or dried cereal	Hockey puck
• 1/2 bagel	
• 1 slice whole-grain bread	

Protein and Dairy	Visual cue
• 2 1/2 ounces chicken or fish	Deck of cards
• 1 1/2 ounces beef	1/2 deck of cards
• 2 ounces hard cheese	4 dice

Fats	Visual cue
• 1 1/2 teaspoons peanut butter	2 dice
• 1 teaspoon butter or margarine	1 die

Recommended daily servings

Once you've established a daily calorie goal — for example, 1,200 calories a day — you can monitor your food intake by sticking to the number of servings recommended for that level. Recommended servings for common daily calorie goals are listed on the bottom of this page.

These servings are spread out over several meals and snacks during the course of your day. If you eat the recommended number of servings, you should be getting about the right number of calories to meet your weight goal. You don't have to count calories, except for when you eat sweets.

The recommended numbers of servings from the carbohydrates, protein and dairy, and fats groups are limits — you shouldn't exceed them. Servings from the vegetables and fruits groups, on the other hand, are minimums. You should eat at least the recommended number of fresh vegetables and fruits listed for your

calorie level. There's no worry if you exceed them.

This premise, however, does not apply to dried fruit, such as raisins and dates, or to fruit juice. These items are higher in energy density, and unlimited servings could cause a significant increase in daily calories.

Avoiding hidden calories

Hidden calories refer to the extra calories in dishes that come from ingredients you may be unaware of. Or you may be aware of them but believe, mistakenly, that they'll have no caloric impact. That's why hidden calories become such a problem for many people grappling with weight control.

Ingredients are often added to enhance the flavor, color or texture of food — for example, seasonings or sauces. Or, ingredients may be added during preparation — for example, oil or butter for frying. These extra calories add up.

- Select appetizers that contain vegetables, fruit or fish. Avoid ones that are fried or breaded.
- Stick with broth-based or tomato-based soups. Avoid creamed or puréed soups and chowders, which can contain heavy cream or egg yolks.
- Choose a simple lettuce or spinach salad with a low-fat dressing. Limit add-ons such as cheese and croutons. Chef salads and taco salads are high-calorie options because of the meat, cheese and other extras — such as the taco salad's shell.
- For side dishes, choose a baked potato, boiled new potatoes, steamed vegetables or rice.
- Look for entrees that are baked, broiled, grilled, roasted, steamed or sautéed in a small amount of oil, broth or water. Avoid items that have been breaded, broasted, creamed, fried or sautéed in heavy oil. Skip pasta dishes with cheese or dishes with sauces containing butter, cream or eggs.

Daily serving recommendations for calorie goals

Food group	Daily calorie goals				
	1,200	1,400	1,600	1,800	2,000
Vegetables	4 or more	4 or more	5 or more	5 or more	5 or more
Fruits	3 or more	4 or more	5 or more	5 or more	5 or more
Carbohydrates	4	5	6	7	8
Protein/Dairy	3	4	5	6	7
Fats	3	3	3	4	5
Sweets	75 calories a day ▶				

Limiting how much you eat

In addition to being aware of serving sizes, other strategies can help you control the amount of food you eat.

- **Eat slowly.** Quick eating creates a time lag between when you stop eating and when your brain registers that you're full. That makes it easy to overeat before you feel the consequences.

- **See what you eat.** Eating directly from a container gives you no sense of serving size. Put your food on a plate or in a bowl.

- **Try to eat three meals at regular times.** Skipping a meal during the day can cause extreme hunger, which can lead to snacking. It's hard to limit how much you eat when you snack.

- **Dish up smaller portions.** At the start of a meal, take slightly less than what you think you'll eat. You can always have seconds, if necessary.

- **Focus on your food.** Avoid distractions. Meals eaten with the television on or while you're reading can lead to mindless eating.

- **Don't feel obligated to clean your plate.** Stop eating as soon as your stomach feels full. Those extra bites of food that you're trying not to waste by cleaning your plate add unneeded calories.

- **Share a meal.** As generous as most restaurant portions are, you and a dining companion may be able to divide a single entree from the menu and satisfy both your appetites.

- **Ask for a carryout bag.** At a restaurant, ask that a portion of your meal be boxed up to take home.

- **Nibble wisely.** If you're still hungry after you've finished eating, instead of refilling your plate, nibble on something low in calories.

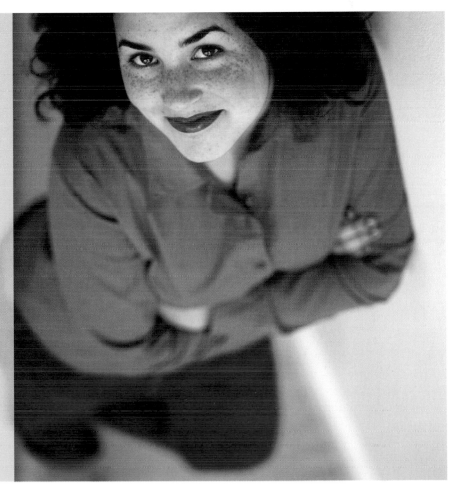

Dietary don'ts

- Don't starve yourself. Try to eat regular meals. If you're hungry between meals, eat. Select most foods from the base of the Healthy Weight Pyramid — vegetables and fruits.

- Don't try to be perfect. You can learn from your mistakes.

- Don't let the occasional setbacks weaken your commitment to lose weight — expect them and know you can get past them.

- Don't be on a timeline. Changing lifelong behaviors is a gradual process and doesn't happen overnight.

- Don't give up — you can do it! Persistence is what carries you through difficult times.

Assess your fitness

Your body burns calories when you're physically active, helping to balance the calories you acquire from the food you eat. To improve your health and lose weight, you want to burn more calories than you take in.

At the most basic level, physical activity means moving — every motion of your body burns calories. Cleaning the house, making the bed, shopping, mowing, gardening, swimming, dancing and playing a pickup game of basketball — these are all forms of physical activity.

Exercise is a structured and repetitive form of physical activity that you do on a regular basis. Exercise improves your fitness, as well as helps you lose weight and deal with everyday stress.

No more excuses

For many people, the mere thought of exercise brings bad memories of high school gym class. You may find yourself besieged with negative thoughts: "It's too hard," "I'm not athletic," "I'm too uncoordinated." Such thoughts are normal, but they don't have to be the final word.

You can become more physically active, but it has to be something you want to do for yourself. If you're doing it for someone else, you likely won't stick with it.

Your odds of sticking with an activity program are generally greater if you:

- **Set realistic goals.** If you start too fast, you'll get frustrated and give up.

- **Choose activities you enjoy.** Not ones you dread.
- **Identify barriers that keep you from exercising.** These might be boredom or lack of time. Try to find solutions for them.

If you find that you're unfit, don't fret. Even the most inactive people can gain considerable health benefits by adding just a few minutes more of physical activity each day.

Adding activity to your day

Take advantage of every chance you have to get up and move around:

- Take the stairs instead of the elevator or escalator.
- Walk or bike to nearby destinations instead of always driving.
- Get off the bus early or park three blocks from work and walk the rest of the way.
- Exercise while watching television, especially during commercials.
- Hide your remote control and get up to change TV channels or adjust the volume.
- If you have a cordless phone, walk around the house while you talk.
- Go for a short walk before breakfast and after dinner.
- Take the dog for a walk.
- Busy yourself with housework, such as vacuuming or washing the windows.
- Work in the garden or yard.
- Wash your car rather than use the automatic carwash.
- Participate in your kids' activities at a playground or park.
- Walk inside instead of use restaurant drive-throughs.
- At the mall, park your car at the far end of the parking lot.

Are you ready for more?

As you think about getting more active, take into account your personal fitness level. Tailor your expectations to your personal situation. You likely can become more active if you're able to:

- Carry out daily tasks without getting overly tired

- Walk a mile or climb a few flights of stairs without becoming winded or feeling heaviness or fatigue in your legs

- Carry on a conversation during moderate exercise, such as taking a brisk walk

When you're not physically active, you become unfit (deconditioned). Signs of deconditioning include feeling tired much of the time and fatiguing quickly. You're unable to keep up with others your age and you avoid certain activities because you know you'll soon tire.

The lean and the restless

You can burn calories in one of two ways. One is to go to the gym and exercise. The other is through all of the activities you do during a normal day. And it appears that daily activity — known as non-exercise activity thermogenesis, or NEAT — is more powerful than is formal exercise when it comes to determining who's lean and who's overweight.

In one of the most detailed and data-rich studies on obesity ever performed, Mayo Clinic researchers found that people who move more during the day — including fidgeting, tapping their toes, wiggling and changing postures — are less likely to gain weight than are people who move less.

Researchers found that some people have a built-in mechanism for keeping weight off through their everyday movements. People who fidget or move around a lot burn extra calories. To the contrary, people who move less burn less. Mayo Clinic researchers found that people who are obese sit, on average, 150 minutes more each day than do their naturally lean counterparts. This means obese people burn 350 fewer calories a day than do lean people.

James Levine, M.D., the Mayo Clinic endocrinologist who led the study, says that people who are obese have a low NEAT, which means they have a bio-

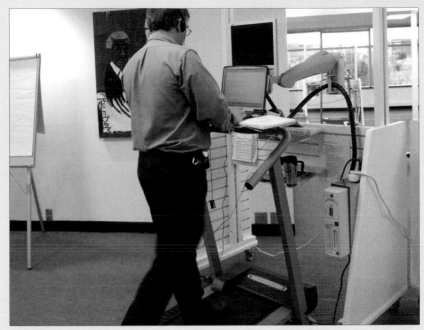

A staff member at work in the Office of the Future.

logical need to sit more. Low NEAT, he emphasizes, doesn't reflect a lack of motivation. "It most likely reflects a brain chemical difference," says Dr. Levine, "because our study shows that even when obese people lose weight, they remain seated the same number of minutes a day. They don't stand or walk more. And conversely, when lean people artificially gain weight, they don't sit more."

This doesn't mean that a person's NEAT can't be altered. Dr. Levine says that in treating individuals who are obese the focus should be not only on food but also on NEAT-seeking behaviors — in other words, moving more.

The message here — whether you're at a healthy weight or you're overweight or obese — is that every calorie you burn by moving counts. Even browsing in a store takes twice

as much energy as does sitting in a chair.

To put his words into action, Dr. Levine has designed what he calls the Office of the Future. In his office, Levine and his colleagues work at treadmills instead of desks. Their computers are stationed on platforms above treadmills, and as they keyboard, they walk. A track encircles the perimeter of the office. When staff want to talk, they take a stroll. Walls near the track are magnetic white boards (instead of fabric) for posting notes and scribbling ideas during the moving meetings.

Dr. Levine says his NEAT office can be modified to any work need and easily constructed in a short time. He believes the cost of the renovation will be paid many times over by the benefits of a healthier staff.

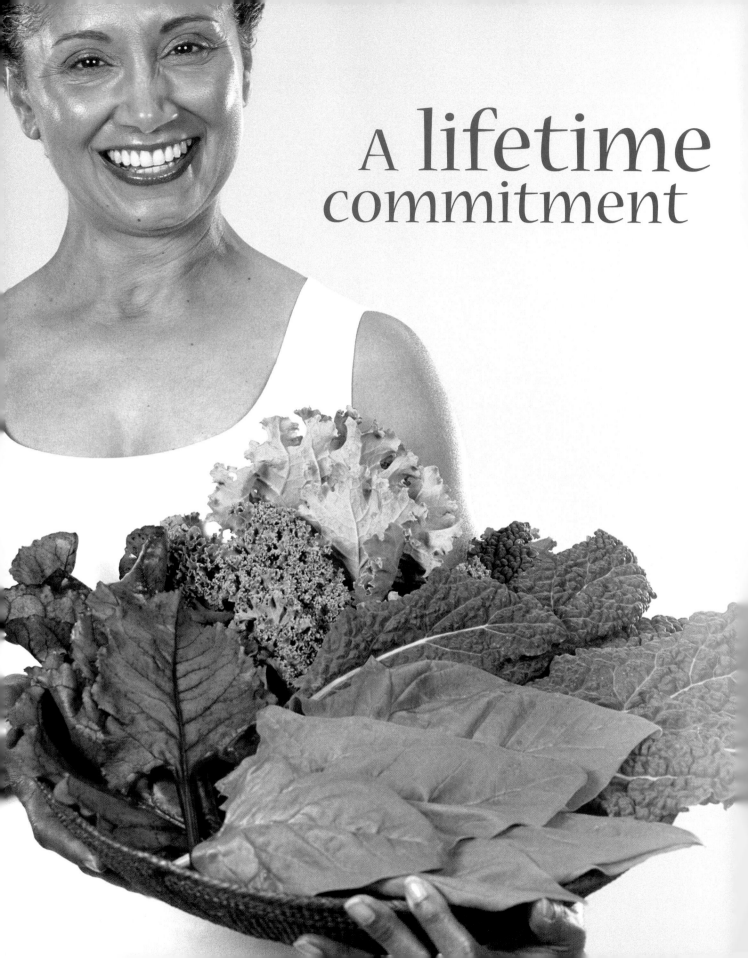

A lifetime
commitment

How often do you find yourself putting food into your mouth when you're not hungry? This question relates to your behavior. Behavior is the way you react to specific situations or to changes in your environment.

Many behaviors that you may feel you were born with are actually ones you've learned over time. For example, newborn babies are remarkably direct when it comes to eating. When they're hungry, they cry for food. When they're full, they refuse to take in a drop more.

You probably don't act that way now. Chances are that over time you've learned eating habits in response to factors other than hunger, factors often triggered by a preoccupied brain rather than an empty stomach. The same thing goes for activity. How active you are is the result of practices you may have learned from your parents or friends.

Anyone who's overweight and who has tried to follow the formula for a healthy weight — eat less and move more — knows it's more challenging than it sounds. What gets in the way? Often, it's learned behaviors — behaviors that have become hard-to-break habits. The good news is that these behaviors can also be unlearned over time.

Many factors — among them emotions, social pressure and lack of awareness — influence behaviors. It's these factors, in addition to what you eat, that you need to target.

Your diet and behavior are integral parts of who you are. If you want to make everlasting changes, it's important to address all aspects of your life.

Preparing to change

Changing a behavior is a highly individualized process. Because everyone's needs are so different and environments so complex, the method, timing and pace of change varies greatly from one person to the next.

As you evaluate your behaviors and take steps to change some of them, here are general principles that may guide you:

- **It's not a race.** The first rule of change is to not change too quickly. A new lifestyle doesn't happen overnight. It takes time and effort to let go of unhealthy behaviors.

- **Forget the scale.** Don't use daily fluctuations of the bathroom scale as a measure of your success. You can control what you eat and what you do more than you can control the numbers. So concentrate on those actions as your goal.

- **Anticipate a lapse.** There will be days when you eat more or move less than you had intended. That's what's called a lapse, and it's inevitable that you'll occasionally lapse. But it's important not to use a lapse as an excuse to give up. Have a plan for such occasions. Keep in mind that a healthy weight results from long-term commitment, not from a single event.

What are your eating triggers?

Think about the times when you've found yourself overeating. Were you eating because you were hungry, or were you eating in response to a feeling or emotion? For many people, food is a coping tool.

Many factors can trigger overeating. Take a few minutes to consider what might be your triggers.

- **Time of day.** Are there certain times of the day when you're more susceptible to overeating?

- **Emotions.** Do you find that certain feelings cause you to snack endlessly?

- **Activities.** Is reading the newspaper or sitting in front of the television a problem without food in your hand?

- **Social situations.** Have you noticed that you eat more around certain people?

- **Foods.** Do you find that the sight or smell of certain foods tempts you to eat?

- **Physical factors.** When you're fatigued, do you turn to junk food as a source of energy? If you have chronic pain, do you use food to distract you from the pain?

How to change a behavior

Behavior change doesn't happen by accident. If you want to make lasting changes in your lifestyle, you need a plan.

There are many strategies for how to change an unhealthy behavior. Everyone has his or her own approach and his or her own pace for making change. And it's likely that you won't follow the same plan for every problem you face. What's important is that you identify and examine those behaviors that interfere with your ability to lose weight and find healthy ways to deal with them.

Following is a list of steps that you may take to change an unhealthy behavior into a healthy one:

1.) List those behaviors that you feel are unhealthy. Common examples include eating too quickly, snacking throughout the day instead of eating regular meals, and skipping your walk when the weather's not perfect or if the television beckons.

2.) Select one behavior that you would like to change and focus only on that one. Trying to change more than one behavior at a time can feel overwhelming and increase the chance that you won't be successful.

3.) Consider how you developed this one behavior. Are there underlying causes that need to be addressed? For example, is all-day snacking related to constant stress?

4.) Think of ways to change this behavior. Come up with several strategies, then decide on one that you feel is practical and doable. Locking yourself out of the kitchen is one way to prevent snacking, but it isn't realistic. Taking time over your noon hour to eat a healthy lunch and to exercise is more realistic.

5.) Devise ways to promote this strategy. How will you go about making time to eat and exercise during a busy day? One option may be to reserve 30 minutes every day over the lunch hour for yourself — when nothing is scheduled.

6.) Make contingency plans for any potential conflicts that might interfere, for example, exercising in the morning before work if you can't avoid a midday meeting.

7.) Set a date for when you would like to achieve your goal. Establish a comfortable pace. It may take you only a few days to make the change, or it may take weeks or months.

8.) When you reach the goal date, evaluate your success. If you didn't reach your goal, what got in the way? Would one of your alternative strategies work better?

9.) Think about what you need to do to make this new behavior a permanent one. If you start letting work responsibilities erode your lunch hour, you'll be back to your old habit of snacking all day.

10.) When ready, select another unhealthy behavior and restart the process. Use the insight you gained from the previous change to help you be successful.

Strategies for change

Here are some general strategies that you may find helpful as you change unhealthy behaviors:

Keep a food record

One of the best ways to understand what causes an unhealthy eating behavior is to keep a food record. In addition to the types and amounts of food you eat, your record may include emotions, social interaction, environment and level of hunger.

Start your record without altering your regular routine. After several days, you may be able to discern behaviors that affect your weight. Whatever the patterns, you can work on changing them.

Have a meal plan

Try to plan your meals at least one day in advance. Planning ahead means the ingredients are on hand and you can start food preparation without delay.

Planning also means packing lunches, snacks or even breakfasts to take to work. This saves you from relying on fast-food fare and making impulsive food choices.

Of course, the best plans can go astray. Have something ready that's healthy to munch on, such as low-calorie popcorn, cut-up vegetables or fruit. This helps if unexpected deadlines or errands interrupt lunch or dinner.

A shopping list is also part of the plan. Following a list helps keep you from impulse buying. Avoid shopping when you're hungry — you'll be tempted to grab anything that looks vaguely appetizing.

Don't tempt yourself

You might trick yourself into believing that bag of chocolate-covered peanuts in the cupboard is for a special occasion. But can you resist sampling them? Do yourself a favor. Don't buy high-calorie foods that tempt you.

That doesn't mean you have to give up sweets and junk food entirely. Just consider not having them in your home. Or store tempting foods out of sight. Where and how you store high-calories foods can influence how much of them you eat.

Keep in mind that as you acquire new eating habits, your tastes will change. Foods that once seemed dreamy eventually may taste too sweet or too fatty. Believe it or not, you can unacquire a taste.

Stick to a schedule

This doesn't necessarily mean the traditional three meals of breakfast, lunch and dinner. You can create a convenient schedule that enables you to eat when you're hungry — perhaps six mini-meals suits you better.

The important thing is you want to avoid constantly snacking throughout the day.

Eat at the table

Designate one place in your home for eating, preferably at a dining room or kitchen table. By eating in one location, you begin to associate that place, and that place only, with food. Even if you're eating by yourself, set the table and make the environment as pleasant as possible.

If you sit in the recliner in the living room and watch television while eating your meals, whenever you sit in the recliner and turn on the television you'll get a craving for food. It's that simple. And it's that difficult. You still may want to eat while watching television, but as you slowly change this bad habit the urge to eat will lessen and should disappear.

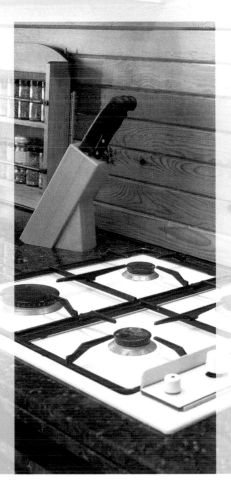

Stop when you're full

Brace yourself for a shock: No matter what your parents told you as a child, you don't have to finish all the food on your plate. Eat slowly and once you begin to feel full, stop. As you become more adept at identifying when you're hungry and when you're satisfied, it becomes easier not to overeat.

Reorganize your kitchen

The kitchen is an obvious place to consider when you're thinking about behaviors that affect weight. Your primary goal is to create a work space that allows you to prepare healthy meals in a short amount of time. This can reduce situations in which you eat unhealthy food because you didn't have the right ingredients handy or you were in a hurry.

Start by replacing the cookie jar with a bowl of fruit. Having a supply of healthy snacks on hand and in plain sight is a good first step. Next, try to keep a good supply of healthy staples in stock — foods and ingredients you use often. While some staples are fairly standard — for example, oatmeal, rice and seasonings — your list will vary, depending on your personal tastes and your talent for cooking.

An efficient kitchen also requires tools. This doesn't mean buying expensive gadgets, just a few high-quality basics will do. Create work areas for specific tasks and keep tools that you use for these tasks nearby. For example, store knives and cutting boards in the food preparation area, and bowls and measuring cups in the mixing area.

Eating out

A trip to the restaurant can be a minefield of temptations. Your best intentions crumble in the company of family and friends as you face all sorts of delicious menu items to chose from. In fact, most everywhere you go these days, the sights and smells of food tantalize your senses: the supermarket deli, the bakery tray at the convenience store, the food court at the mall, the concession stand at the theater.

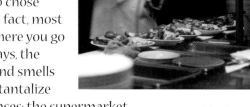

For many people, eating out is common practice. They choose to do so because it's convenient, efficient and fun. Eating out is also a factor commonly associated with weight gain. That's why you can't let your guard down at the restaurant or snack bar, especially if you eat there often.

Does that mean you can't leave the house if you want to eat healthy? Not at all. You just need to be aware of healthy choices. You should also be mindful of two common dining-out challenges: the urge to order more food than you need and the impulse to eat every bit of food on your plate — even when the portions are too large.

- Eat slowly and savor each bite. When you begin to feel full, stop eating. If you have food left, ask for a takeout box or doggie bag and take it home for another meal.
- Eat foods that are healthy and low in calories first. You can eat a lot of these foods — so when it's time to enjoy a higher calorie food, you won't be so hungry.

- Portion sizes in restaurants can be two to three times the amount you need. If you receive large portions, eat only half and save the rest.

- Limit other items you eat before or during your meal, such as appetizers, bread, side dishes and high-calorie beverages.
- Look for ways to make your entree more healthy. For example, if your favorite dish comes with a rich sauce, ask for the sauce on the side and don't eat it all. Ask if the item can be broiled instead of fried.
- Don't stand next to or sit near the hors d'oeuvre table or buffet line. As the saying goes, "Out of sight, out of mind."
- Finish your main meal before ordering dessert. By the time you're done, you may not want dessert. If you do, consider splitting it with one of your companions. Some healthy options include sorbet and sherbet.
- If you know that you'll be eating out, increase your exercise for that day.
- Eat something healthy a short time before going out. If you arrive at the restaurant hungry, you'll be more inclined to overeat.

When you're traveling

It may be a bit more difficult to eat healthy when you're traveling, but it's certainly not impossible. The rules for healthy eating at a neighborhood restaurant still apply when you're in a restaurant farther from home.

Difficulties generally stem from the fast pace of travel and from your unfamiliarity with the healthy options that are available in a new place. It's always best if you can be well-informed about the locations you're visiting and anticipate problems.

Avoid rationalizations such as, "I'm traveling, so I'll have to eat whatever is available."

- If you travel by car, pack a cooler with healthy foods, such as sandwiches, yogurt, fruit and raw vegetables.
- If you travel by plane, pack snacks such as nuts and fruit in your carry-on bag.
- Stay hydrated while you travel by drinking plenty of calorie-free beverages. That includes coffee, hot tea, calorie-free iced tea and diet soda. But water is the best choice!
- If you have free time between flights, tour the airport terminal to see what healthy restaurant options are available. Look for fresh garden salads, fresh fruit, baked potatoes, vegetable pizza or sandwich wraps, grilled chicken sandwiches and pasta entrees in tomato sauce.

- Ask hotel employees about restaurants that have healthy options on their menus, or that offer grilled or broiled foods. You might also ask if there's a grocery store nearby where you can purchase fruit and easy-to-fix items.

- If food cravings strike, try to distract yourself. Telephone a friend, inspect the exercise facilities at the place where you're staying or go for a walk. When your mind is occupied with something else, the cravings quickly go away.

- At business events, use portion control. Allow yourself small servings of some higher calorie foods so that you don't feel deprived, but eat larger servings of foods that are lower in calories.

- Focus your mind on the benefits of eating healthy and on how it will give you the energy you need for your trip.

Assessing the salad bar

When dining out, you may think that choosing the salad bar is a healthy alternative to ordering from the menu. However, unless you make careful choices, you could end up with a plate filled with calories and fat.

Before ordering, walk along the salad bar to see if it has the ingredients you like for a tasty, healthy salad. Some salad bars look more like a delicatessen, with a lot of rich, high-fat choices. Remember that just because a food is located in the salad bar doesn't automatically mean that it's healthy.

- **Examine the greens.** Lettuce or spinach is generally the foundation of a healthy salad. Do the greens look crisp and fresh?

- **Survey the fresh vegetables and fruits.** In addition to greens, you may want to pile on tomatoes, mushrooms, carrots, broccoli, cauliflower, cucumbers, beets, bell peppers, pineapple, cantaloupe, grapes and strawberries. Is there a varied offering of these items?

- **Be wary of the extras.** Many people go wrong at salad bars by including too many high fat ingredients, such as cheese, chopped eggs, bacon bits and buttery croutons. Beware of other types of salads such as pasta salad or potato salad. Can you use the salad bar and take only very small amounts of these items or avoid them all together?

- **Don't forget the dressings.** Look for fat-free or low-fat, low-calorie versions. Other options include vinegars. You can also add flavor to your salad with herbs and peppers.

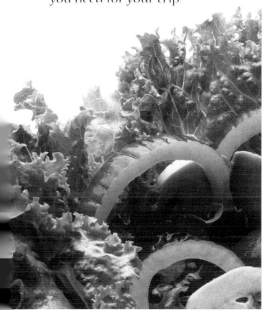
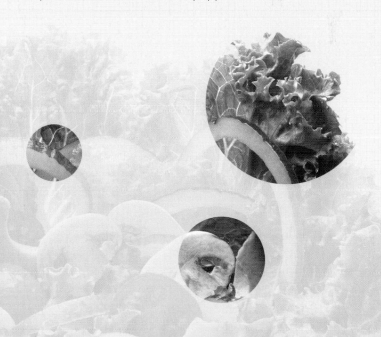

Bumps in the road

It's the million-dollar question. How do you maintain a lifelong commitment to weight control? If this question had an easy answer, nearly everyone would be at a healthy weight.

The truth is, maintaining a healthy weight is challenging. Even if you're committed for the long haul for all of the right reasons, your resolve will be tested time and again. How you respond can be the difference between weight-loss success or failure.

Plateaus

There's no greater reward than to step on the bathroom scale and see that you've lost weight.

But what happens when the scale doesn't change from week to week? Even if you're eating a healthy, low-calorie diet and exercising regularly — by all accounts, doing everything right — the results aren't showing up. Days may go by, even weeks, when your weight remains unchanged. You've reached what's known as a plateau.

Before you get discouraged, understand that the long-term results of a weight program take time. If your program has stalled, make sure you're on track with weight-loss basics. One of these suggestions may help:

- Assess your food and activity records. Have you loosened the rules, letting yourself get by with larger portions or less exercise?
- Focus on three- to four-week trends instead of daily fluctu-

ations. You may find that, even if progress is not evident immediately, you're still losing weight.

- Remain positive. Remember that results aren't measured in pounds alone. Find other ways in which your health has improved.

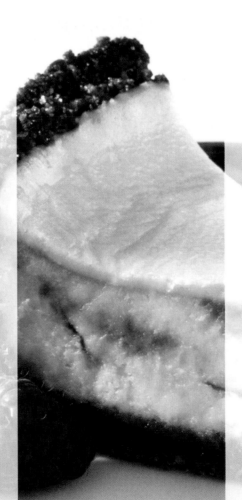

If you feel that you've truly hit a plateau, it's time to reassess your program. You may have lost all the weight that you will lose based on your calorie and exercise goals.

At this point, you need to ask yourself if you can be happy with the weight you're at. If you want to lose additional pounds, you'll need to adjust your program.

- Reduce your daily calorie intake by 200 calories — provided this doesn't put you below 1,200 calories a day. Too few calories may cause you to feel hungry all of the time and increase the risk of binge eating.

- Gradually increase the amount of time you exercise by an additional 15 to 30 minutes. You may also increase the intensity of your exercise, if you feel that's possible. Additional exercise will cause you to burn more calories.

- Aside from exercise, increase your daily physical activity. For example, use your car less or plan to do more yardwork.

- If you find these changes difficult, re-examine your weight-loss goal. Maybe the weight you're striving for is unrealistic for you.

- Don't throw in the towel. Just because weight loss is now more difficult, don't revert back to your old habits. That may cause you to regain all of the weight you've lost.

Behavior chains

It's happened to everyone. You're having a good day — you ate fresh fruit at breakfast, biked to work and took a 15-minute walk during your lunch break. Then a midafternoon craving sends you sprinting for the vending machine. Minutes later, you're back at your desk with a candy bar in hand.

What happened? Maybe you were tired, or you didn't eat enough at lunch. Whatever the reason, you let a craving get the best of you. Now you're upset and angry — feelings that may send you back to the vending machine.

Imagine these events as a chain of separate but interconnected behaviors. Try to separate this chain into discrete parts.

Take the example of a woman named Laura, who lets an unfortunate chain of behaviors sabotage her eating plan:

- Laura agrees to bring cookies to a friend's potluck dinner.
- She buys the cookies two days beforehand.
- She works late and misses lunch.
- Laura arrives home very hungry.
- She thinks, "I'll eat one cookie, then go to the grocery store."
- She takes the box of cookies to the den.
- Laura starts eating cookies while watching television and reading her mail.
- She eats rapidly and without awareness.
- She feels guilty and eats more.
- Laura dumps her eating plan.

At every link, Laura could have done something to break the chain of events. She could have agreed to bring a salad or a type of dessert she doesn't crave. She could have waited until the day of the party to buy the cookies. Knowing that missing lunch is risky, she could have set aside 15 minutes to order a carryout salad from a nearby restaurant. She could have taken one or two cookies into the den, not the entire box. Finally, she could have convinced herself that this incident was just a lapse and that she should continue her weight program.

You can do the same with your behavior chains. Try interrupting a chain at the earliest link. If a midafternoon craving regularly strikes, you may break the chain by stocking your office desk with healthy snacks. Or maybe you can plan a healthy dinner before leaving for work, and have the ingredients on hand when you arrive home. Self control is easier to exercise than willpower. Don't lead yourself into temptation.

Lapse and relapse

Rare is the person who doesn't experience a lapse from time to time. Whether it's sneaking dessert after an already decadent meal or missing a daily walk, lapses are bound to happen. Danger occurs when lapses turn into relapses.

What's the difference? A lapse happens when you revert to old behaviors once or twice. It's temporary, common and a sign that you need to get back in control.

A relapse is more serious. When several lapses occur within a short span of time, you're at risk of reverting back to your old behavior. It might happen during a vacation when weight control takes a back seat, or during a busy week at work when you can't eat or exercise as you'd hoped.

Often, you panic. You say, "I guess I just can't do it." That helps trigger the relapse. You're giving up on weight control. Relapse is what you must avoid.

When you experience a lapse, the best thing you can do is to calm down and see the situation for what it is: normal and temporary. Also consider these tips:

- Don't let negative thoughts take over. Remember that mistakes happen and that each day is a chance to start anew.

- Clearly identify the problem, then think of possible solutions. If a solution works, then you've got yourself a plan for preventing another lapse. If it doesn't work, try another solution until you find one that works.

- Guilt from the initial lapse often leads to more lapses. Being prepared and having a plan is important for overcoming guilt.

- Work out your frustration with exercise. Take a walk or

go for a swim. Keep the exercise upbeat. Never use exercise as punishment for a lapse.

• Get support. Talk to a friend or professional counselor.

• Recommit to your goals. Review them and make sure they're still realistic.

What if you do relapse? Although relapses are disappointing, they may help you realize that your goals are unrealistic, or that you're putting yourself in high-risk situations, or that certain strategies don't work for you.

Above all, realize that you're not a failure. Reverting to old behaviors doesn't mean that all hope is lost. It just means that you need to recharge your motivation, recommit to your program and return to healthy behaviors.

Stress

Stress is what you experience when life's demands exceed your ability to cope. A fast-paced environment or change of routine can trigger stress. So can an illness in the family. Or if you get a promotion. Or when the holidays arrive in all their cookie-covered glory.

When stressful situations occur, you may turn to food for comfort. You may lose focus on your exercise routine. Unfortunately, these responses to stress simply create more havoc in your life.

To stay on track through stressful times, consider these strategies:

• Simplify and prioritize your schedule. Deal with only one thing at a time.

• Plan a week's worth of meals ahead of time. Use a grocery list to eliminate last-minute trips to the store.

• Devote time on the weekend to preparing meals for the coming week and freeze them in meal-sized batches.

• Remember that healthy meals don't have to be complicated. Serve a large, fresh salad with fat-free dressing, a whole-grain roll and a piece of fruit.

• Tackle unpleasant tasks early in the day.

• Go to bed 30 minutes earlier at night. Sleep gives you energy to face the next day.

• Have family members help out around the house. Split up the tasks to save time.

• Organize your day to avoid conflicts or last-minute rushes. Delegate some work.

• Be patient. Realize that improvements in your weight and overall health take time.

• Go with the flow. Not every battle has to be fought.

Bolster your body image

A sad fact is that only about one in seven adult Americans is happy with his or her body. Dissatisfaction with body size and shape can cause feelings of disappointment or disgust and trigger overeating and weight gain.

Appreciate the body you have. Write a list of your strengths and your best features.

Make a list of people you most admire. Do they have perfect bodies? Does it matter?

Don't take yourself for granted. Take care of yourself each day. Eat well, be physically active and get plenty of rest.

Get support. Surround yourself with friends who don't focus on body size or appearance.

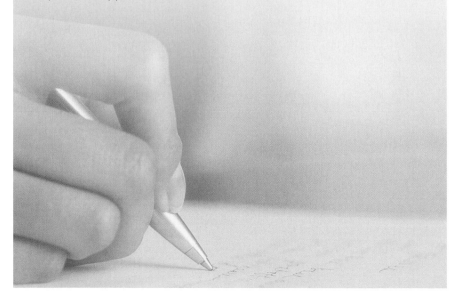

How are you doing?

Are the results so far meeting your expectations? Judging your progress in terms of numbers — your weight when you started the program and your weight at this moment — may make you happy. But it may also lead to disappointment. Many people believe they can never lose enough weight.

Remember that weight control isn't only about the number of pounds you've lost. Consider that you're now eating better and that you're more active. Other measures of success include more energy, improved fitness, better self-image and more positive moods. With weight control, you lower your risk of high blood pressure, high cholesterol, diabetes, cardiovascular disease, osteoarthritis and many types of cancers.

Any weight loss, no matter how small, is a big, healthy step in the right direction. If you feel that you still need to lose more weight, keep going. With all that you've learned, you'll ultimately reach your goal.

Sometimes, a lifetime commitment to weight control depends on your ability to accept your body for what it is, with all of its imperfections (and perfections). The strategies described here can help you develop a healthier body image and boost your self-esteem:

- **Stick to basic principles.** Continue to focus on maintaining a healthy lifestyle, and the weight will take care of itself. Stick with a balanced diet, moderate portions and daily physical activity. Get enough sleep and try to manage your stress level. Remember that these principles apply to everyone, not just people wanting to lose weight.

- **Persistence pays off.** Keep doing whatever has worked for you in the past. Adapt these strategies to new situations. You can vary them or add to them to keep things interesting and challenging. Every step forward, every day, is important.

- **Make it enjoyable.** The things you do to maintain your weight

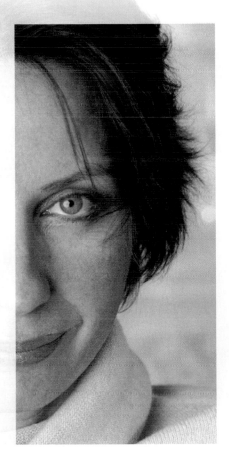

should be things you look forward to doing. You want them to be enjoyable and comforting, not unpleasant, tiresome or boring. Once you start finding excuses or dragging your feet, your new and improved behaviors will be quickly cast aside.

- **Keep a long-term perspective.** Regardless of how many pounds you've lost, the fact that you stayed with the program may be your most important achievement. Your health has improved and your self-esteem is stronger. It's important to consider weight control beyond just a 12-week or 12-month period. It's for a lifetime. And no matter what your expectations are, by staying committed, you'll reach your goal — even if it's a little later than you had planned on.

- **Give yourself credit.** Acknowledge the vital role you've played in your success. It was your commitment to losing weight that got you started. It was your energy and focus that kept you moving through the weeks. You now have the tools and experience to continue on. Taking stock of what you've accomplished and giving yourself credit for those accomplishments helps to improve your confidence level so that you can manage whatever challenges may come along in the future.

Menus and recipes

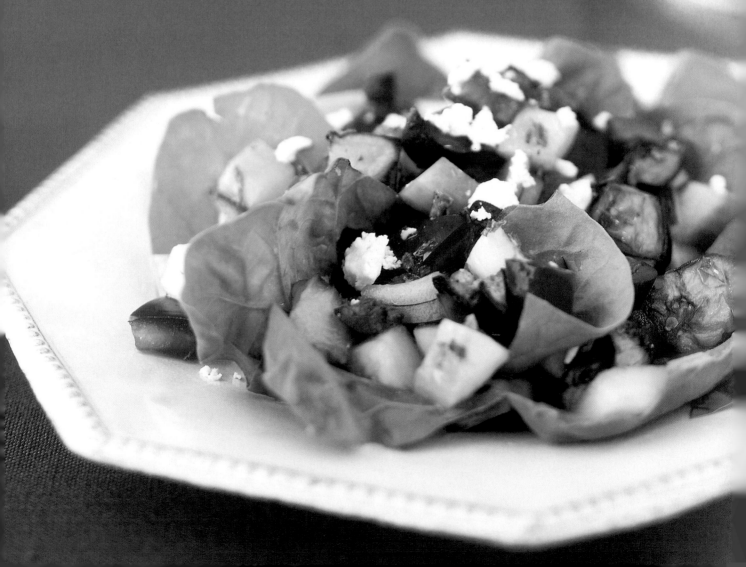

You now have the basic elements for starting the Mayo Clinic Healthy Weight Program:

- You feel that you're motivated and ready.
- You've decided on your weight-loss goals.
- You've determined your daily calorie goal.
- You've determined your daily servings totals from the food groups of the Mayo Clinic Healthy Weight Pyramid.
- You understand you need daily physical activity and you're ready to get active. (If you're out of shape — especially if you have health concerns — see your doctor before beginning the program.)

To help you get started on your path to better eating, on the following pages you'll find a week's worth of menus and recipes. You don't need to follow the menus exactly. It's OK to follow them only partially and substitute your own meals whenever you like. Use the servings lists on pages 119 to 123 to develop your own healthy meals.

If you're worried about being able to select and prepare nutritious meals on your own, don't be. It's not difficult to integrate the Mayo Clinic Healthy Weight Pyramid into your daily diet and to adjust it to suit your tastes. The important thing is to meet your requirements for the daily food servings. For example, with a daily goal of 1,200 calories, aim for at least four vegetable servings and three fruit servings, as well as four carbohydrate servings, three protein and dairy servings and three fat servings.

Kitchen staples

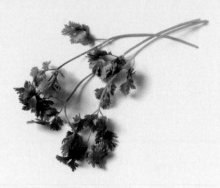

Keep your kitchen stocked with the following ingredients. When you run short of a particular item, add it to your weekly shopping list. You can include other items on your staples list.

Baking powder and baking soda
Beans (kidney and black)
Bouillon cubes (chicken and vegetable)
Breakfast cereal, whole-grain
Cooking spray, vegetable
Corn, frozen
Cornmeal
Cornstarch
Crackers (whole-grain, wheat, saltine)
Croutons, seasoned
Flour, all-purpose
Honey
Jam or jelly, any flavor
Ketchup
Lemon juice
Margarine, trans-fat-free
Mayonnaise, reduced-calorie
Molasses, light
Mustard (regular, Dijon, honey)
Nuts (almonds and peanuts)
Oatmeal
Oil (canola, extra-virgin olive, sesame, peanut)
Pasta, whole-grain (linguine, spaghetti, shells)
Peanut butter
Peas, frozen
Raisins
Rice (brown and wild)
Salad dressings, reduced-calorie
Seeds (sesame and sunflower)
Soy sauce, low-sodium
Stock or broth (chicken and vegetable)
Sugar (brown and white)

Syrup
Tomatoes, canned (diced and whole)
Tomato paste and tomato sauce
Tortilla chips, baked
Tortillas, fat-free (corn or flour)
Tuna, canned, water-packed
Vinegar (balsamic, cider, white and red wine, herb-flavored)
Wine, for cooking (white and red)

Herbs, seasonings and spices (dry)
Basil
Bay leaf
Celery seed
Chili powder
Cinnamon, ground
Cloves, ground
Cumin
Dill weed
Garlic powder
Ginger, ground
Mustard, dry
Onion powder
Oregano
Parsley
Pepper (black, cayenne, garlic and lemon)
Rosemary
Salt
Thyme

Day 1 menu

Breakfast

1 c. reduced-calorie, fat-free yogurt   *P/D* ●

1 large banana   *Fruit* ● ●

Calorie-free beverage

Snack

1 serving favorite fruit   *Fruit* ●

Lunch

Smoked turkey wrap
Carbohydrates ●, *P/D* ●, *Fat* ●

Top a 6-inch tortilla with 3 oz. thin-sliced smoked turkey, shredded lettuce, sliced tomato and onion. Top with 2 tbsp. reduced-calorie Western dressing and roll up.

Cucumber and tomato salad
Vegetables ●

Combine ½ c. thinly sliced cucumber and 4 cherry tomatoes, halved. Add rice wine or herb-flavored vinegar to taste.

Calorie-free beverage

Dinner

1 serving pasta with fresh tomato sauce   *Carbohydrates* ● ●, *Vegetables* ● ● ●, *Fat* ● ●

½ c. fat-free frozen yogurt or fat-free vanilla ice cream *P/D* ●

Calorie-free beverage

Daily recommended servings

Vegetables (no limit) ● ● ● ●   Fruits (no limit) ● ● ●
Carbohydrates ● ● ● ●   Protein & Dairy (P/D) ● ● ●   Fats ● ● ●

Dietitian's tips

- Fresh vegetables generally provide the best texture and taste at meals, but if you don't have access to fresh produce, it's OK to use frozen varieties. Canned vegetables also may be substituted, but watch for added salt or sugar.

- If you don't have fresh herbs on hand, you can use dried herbs instead. Because dried herbs have a more intense flavor, use less of them. Add only one-third to one-half the amount called for. Crush before using to bring out the flavor. These common varieties contribute color, taste and aroma to most dishes:

Basil. An herb with a sweet, clove-like taste, best used with Italian foods, especially tomatoes, tomato sauces, pasta, chicken, fish and shellfish

Caraway. Seeds with a nutty, licorice flavor, best used with cooked vegetables such as beets, cabbage, carrots, potatoes, turnips and winter squash

Chives. A member of the onion family, with long, hollow green stems and a mild onion flavor, best used with sauces, soups, baked potatoes, salads, omelets, pasta, seafood and meat

Dill. An herb with a mild sweet but tangy flavor, best used with seafood, chicken, yogurt, cucumbers, green beans, tomatoes, potatoes and beets

Oregano. An herb with a somewhat sweet and peppery flavor, best used with Italian and Greek cuisine, and meat and poultry dishes

Thyme. An herb with a strong, minty, somewhat bitter flavor, best used with fish, poultry, tomatoes, beans, eggplant, mushrooms and potatoes

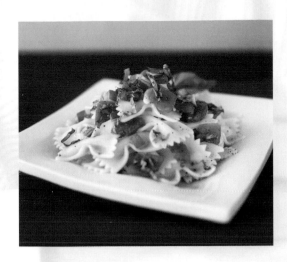

Ingredients list

4 tomatoes, about 2 lbs. total weight, peeled and seeded, and cut into ½-inch cubes

½ c. (¾ oz.) fresh basil, diced, plus whole leaves for garnish

3 tbsp. chopped red onion

3 tbsp. extra-virgin olive oil

1 tbsp. red wine vinegar

1 clove garlic, finely minced

¾ tsp. salt

¼ tsp. freshly ground pepper

½ lb. pasta

Per serving

Calories	372
Protein	10 g
Carbohydrates	58 g
Total fat	12 g
Saturated fat	2 g
Monounsaturated fat	8 g
Cholesterol	0 mg
Sodium	463 mg
Fiber	5 g

Pasta with fresh tomato sauce

Serves: 4

To make the sauce, in a large bowl, combine the tomatoes, basil, onion, olive oil, vinegar, garlic, salt and pepper. Toss gently.

Fill a large pot ¾ full with water and bring to a boil. Add the pasta and cook until al dente, 10-12 minutes, or according to package directions. Drain the pasta thoroughly.

Divide the pasta among warmed individual bowls. Top each serving with sauce and garnish with a fresh basil leaf.

Day 2 menu

Breakfast

½ whole-grain English muffin
or 1 slice whole-grain toast
Carbohydrates ●

1 tbsp. honey

½ large grapefruit
Fruit ●

Calorie-free beverage

Lunch

Southwestern salad
Fruit ●, *Vegetables* ● ●, *P/D* ●,
Fat ● ●

Top 2 c. shredded lettuce with 2½ oz. shredded cooked chicken, 1 c. chopped green bell peppers and onions, ½ c. crushed pineapple, ⅛ avocado, and 2 tbsp. reduced-calorie Western-style salad dressing.

½ whole-grain pita bread
Carbohydrates ●

Calorie-free beverage

Dinner

1 serving Tuscan white bean stew
Vegetables ●, *Carbohydrates* ●,
P/D ● ●

6 whole-grain crackers
Carbohydrates ●

1 c. grapes *Fruit* ●

Calorie-free beverage

Snack

1 serving favorite vegetable
Vegetables ●

2 tbsp. low-calorie vegetable dip
Fat ●

Daily recommended servings

Vegetables (no limit) ● ● ●   Fruits (no limit) ● ● ●
Carbohydrates ● ● ●   Protein & Dairy (P/D) ● ● ●   Fats ● ● ●

Dietitian's tips

- Soup is an easy, nutritious meal. When you don't have enough time to make your own, it's OK to use canned or dried soups. To help keep calories in check, add water or skim milk to soup concentrate. Select soups that are loaded with vegetables.

  - It's OK on occasion to substitute a convenience food for a conventional dinner, especially on those days when you have little time to cook. Convenience foods, such as pizza or frozen entrees, can be healthy, provided you choose wisely. Read the nutrition label on the packages. Look for dishes that have no more than 300 to 450 calories and 5 to 10 grams of fat for the whole meal. Some healthy frozen entrees include chicken chow mein with rice, salisbury steak, vegetarian chili and chicken cacciatore.

- Peppers — there are hundreds of varieties — vary from mild and sweet to fiery hot. They add color, texture, flavor and, depending on the variety, mouth-blistering heat to recipes. The heat comes from the pepper's capsaicin, which is found in its seeds and membranes. Here's the order of peppers from mild to hot: bell peppers (mild and sweet), Anaheim, poblano, jalapeno, serrano, Tabasco, habanero (fire). Chipotle peppers are smoked jalapeno peppers.

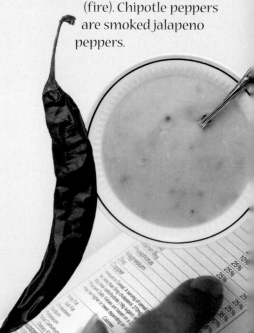

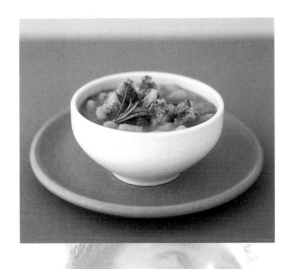

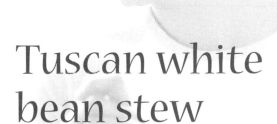

Ingredients list

Croutons
1 tbsp. extra-virgin olive oil
2 cloves garlic, quartered
1 slice (1 oz.) whole-grain bread, cut into ½-inch cubes

Soup
2 c. (14 oz.) dried cannellini or other white beans, rinsed, soaked overnight, and drained
6 c. (48 fl. oz.) water
1 tsp. salt
1 bay leaf
2 tbsp. olive oil
1 yellow onion, coarsely chopped
3 carrots, peeled and coarsely chopped
6 cloves garlic, chopped
¼ tsp. freshly ground pepper
1 tbsp. chopped fresh rosemary, plus 6 sprigs
1½ c. (12 fl. oz.) vegetable stock or broth

Per serving

Calories	328
Protein	15 g
Carbohydrates	51 g
Total fat	8 g
Saturated fat	1 g
Monounsaturated fat	5 g
Cholesterol	0 mg
Sodium	423 mg
Fiber	19 g

Tuscan white bean stew

Serves: 6

To make the croutons, in a large frying pan, heat the olive oil over medium heat. Add the garlic and sauté for 1 minute. Remove from the heat and let stand for 10 minutes to infuse the garlic flavor into the oil. Remove the garlic and discard. Return the pan to medium heat. Add the bread cubes and sauté, stirring frequently, until lightly browned, 3-5 minutes. Transfer to a small bowl and set aside.

In a soup pot over high heat, combine the white beans, water, ½ tsp. of the salt and the bay leaf. Bring to a boil over high heat. Reduce the heat to low, cover partially, and simmer until the beans are tender, 60-75 minutes. Drain the beans, reserving ½ c. (4 fl. oz.) of the cooking liquid. Discard the bay leaf.

In a small bowl, combine the reserved cooking liquid and ½ c. (3½ oz.) of the cooked beans. Mash with a fork to form a paste. Stir the bean paste into the cooked beans.

Return the pot to the stove and add the olive oil. Heat over medium-high heat. Stir in the onion and carrots and sauté until the carrots are tender-crisp, 6-7 minutes. Stir in the garlic and cook until softened, about 1 minute. Stir in the remaining ½ tsp. salt, the pepper, the chopped rosemary, the bean mixture and the stock. Bring to a boil, then reduce the heat to low and simmer until the stew is heated through, about 5 minutes.

Ladle into individual bowls and sprinkle with the croutons. Garnish each bowl with a rosemary sprig.

Day 3 menu

Breakfast

½ c. whole-grain cereal
Carbohydrates ●

½ c. skim milk *P/D* ●

1 small banana or 1 medium orange *Fruit* ●

Calorie-free beverage

Lunch

Chef salad *Vegetables* ● ● , *P/D* ●

Top 2 c. mixed greens with 1 oz. low-fat cheddar cheese strips, 1 ½ oz. turkey strips, and 1 c. sliced tomatoes, cucumbers, green peppers, broccoli florets and red onion.

2 tbsp. reduced-calorie French dressing *Fat* ●

6 whole-grain crackers
Carbohydrates ●

Calorie-free beverage

Dinner

1 serving chicken and portobello baguette *Vegetables* ● ● , *Carbohydrates* ● ● , *P/D* ● , *Fat* ● ●

1 small apple *Fruit* ●

Calorie-free beverage

Snack

1 serving favorite fruit *Fruit* ●

Daily recommended servings

Vegetables (no limit) ● ● ● ●
Carbohydrates ● ● ● ●

Fruits (no limit) ● ● ●
Protein & Dairy (P/D) ● ● ●   Fats ● ● ●

Dietitian's tips

- Vary your salad greens to take advantage of the multitude of flavors and textures. There are four basic types. Head lettuce (iceberg) has a crisp texture and mild flavor. Butterhead (Boston or bibb) lettuce is delicate in texture and flavor. Loose-leaf lettuce (red-leaf or green-leaf) has easily separated leaves that are flavorful and crisp. Romaine (cos) lettuce has a crunchy texture and somewhat bitter taste. Try a different variety each week.

- Don't be fooled into thinking "low-calorie" dressings are really low in calories. Most aren't. According to labeling laws, a "low-calorie" salad dressing may have up to 40 calories per serving. When possible, choose fat-free dressings. They generally have 25 calories or less per serving.

- If you're preparing chicken breasts for a meal, why not cook a few extra breasts for upcoming meals? Cooked chicken may be safely used for up to two days, if kept covered and refrigerated. Also, if time is an issue, precooked, packaged chicken breasts can be used in a variety of salads and sandwiches.

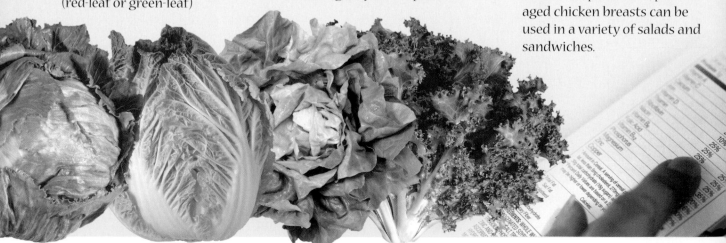

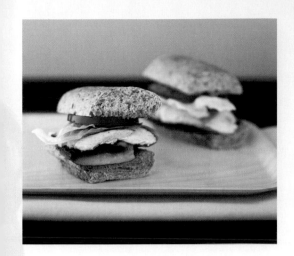

Ingredients list

1 large red bell pepper, roasted
   and seeded
1 shallot, chopped
1½ tbsp. chopped walnuts
1½ tbsp. balsamic vinegar
1 tsp. Dijon mustard
¼ tsp. plus ⅛ tsp. salt
¼ tsp. plus ⅛ tsp. freshly ground
   pepper
2 tbsp. extra-virgin olive oil
¾ lb. skinless, boneless chicken
   breasts
2 large portobello mushrooms,
   stemmed, brushed clean, and
   halved
1 whole-grain baguette, cut
   crosswise into 4 sections, each
   about 6 inches long
4 butterhead (Boston) lettuce
   leaves
1 tomato, thinly sliced

Per serving

Calories	400
Protein	30 g
Carbohydrates	44 g
Total fat	13 g
Saturated fat	2 g
Monounsaturated fat	7 g
Cholesterol	49 mg
Sodium	692 mg
Fiber	8 g

Chicken and portobello baguette

Serves: 4

Chop the roasted bell pepper coarsely. In a blender or food processor, combine the roasted pepper, shallot, walnuts, 1 tbsp. of the vinegar, the mustard, ¼ tsp. of the salt, and ¼ tsp. of the pepper. Pulse a few times to purée and set aside.

In a large, nonstick frying pan, heat 1½ tsp. of the olive oil over medium high heat. Season the chicken breasts with the remaining ⅛ tsp. salt and ⅛ tsp. pepper. Add the chicken to the pan and cook, turning once, until lightly browned on both sides and no longer pink on the inside, 3-4 minutes on each side. Transfer to a cutting board and let cool. Thinly slice the chicken lengthwise into strips.

In the same frying pan, heat the remaining 1½ tbsp. olive oil over medium-high heat. Add the mushrooms and sauté, turning frequently, until well browned, 7-9 minutes. Remove from the heat and drizzle with the remaining 1½ tsp. balsamic vinegar.

Cut the baguette sections in half lengthwise. Spread about 1 tbsp. red pepper mixture on both halves of each baguette section. Place 1 mushroom half on the bottom baguette section. Top with ¼ of the chicken, a lettuce leaf, and 1 or 2 tomato slices. Close the sandwich with the top half of the baguette section, and slice in half. Repeat to make 3 more sandwiches (If making ahead, omit the red pepper mixture, wrap the sandwiches in plastic wrap, and refrigerate. Spread the red pepper mixture on the baguettes just before serving.)

Day 4 menu

Breakfast

Omelet *Vegetables* ●, *P/D* ●

Mix ½ c. egg substitute with ½ c. diced onions, tomatoes, green peppers and mushrooms, and cook until set.

1 slice whole-grain toast *Carbohydrates* ●

1 tsp. margarine *Fat* ●

1 small banana *Fruit* ●

Calorie-free beverage

Lunch

California burger *Vegetables* ●, *Carbohydrates* ● ●, *P/D* ● ●, *Fat* ●

Top 3 oz. cooked extra-lean ground beef patty or vegetable burger with ½ grilled onion, lettuce and tomato slices. Serve on a small whole-grain bun spread with 1 tbsp. reduced-calorie mayonnaise.

1 small apple *Fruit* ●

Calorie-free beverage

Dinner

1 serving Greek salad *Vegetables* ● ●, *Fat* ●

6 whole-grain crackers *Carbohydrates* ●

Calorie-free beverage

Snack

1 serving favorite fruit *Fruit* ●

Daily recommended servings Vegetables (no limit) ● ● ● ●   Fruits (no limit) ● ● ●
Carbohydrates ● ● ● ●   Protein & Dairy (P/D) ● ● ●   Fats ● ● ●

Dietitian's tips

A good piece of fresh fruit, in particular, is the ideal snack — it's low in calories, satisfying and healthy. Here are suggestions for different ways that you can enjoy vegetables and fruits as snacks:

- Make a fruit smoothie by blending fruit with low-fat yogurt or skim milk.
- Cut fruit in slices or halves and dip the pieces in low-fat cottage cheese or yogurt.
- Make frozen fruit chips. Purée fruit and then freeze it.
- Freeze fresh grapes and enjoy them in warm weather.

- Use chunks of fresh fruit to make fruit kebabs on skewers.
- Dip partially cooked vegetables (carrots, green beans, broccoli, cauliflower) in cottage cheese, hummus, low-fat ranch dressing or yogurt dip.
- Lightly spread peanut butter or low-fat cream cheese on bell pepper slices, zucchini chunks or tomato wedges.
- Spread peanut butter on celery slices and top the peanut butter with raisins.
- Mix low-fat ricotta cheese with unsweetened pineapple and spread on celery strips.

- Make vegetable kebabs with bell pepper strips, mushrooms, cherry tomatoes and zucchini chunks.

Other kinds of food offer snack options. Nuts are a good choice as long as the portion size is reasonable — a little goes a long way in terms of making you feel full. Different kinds of brown-rice and wild-rice cakes are low in calories. Some whole-grain crackers and cereal fit the bill as well.

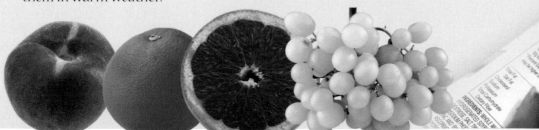

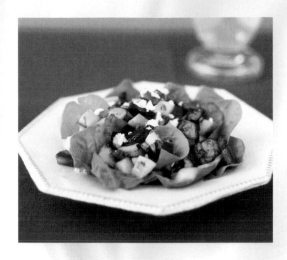

Ingredients list

Vinaigrette
1 tbsp. red wine vinegar
1 tbsp. fresh lemon juice
2 tsp. chopped fresh oregano or ¾ tsp. dried oregano
½ tsp. salt
¼ tsp. freshly ground pepper
2½ tbsp. extra-virgin olive oil

Salad
1 large eggplant, about 1 ½ lb., trimmed and cut into ½-inch cubes
1 lb. spinach, stemmed and torn into bite-sized pieces
1 cucumber, peeled, seeded, and diced
1 tomato, seeded and diced
½ red onion, diced
2 tbsp. pitted, chopped black Greek olives
2 tbsp. crumbled feta cheese

Per serving

Calories	88
Protein	3 g
Carbohydrates	9 g
Total fat	5 g
Saturated fat	1 g
Monounsaturated fat	3 g
Cholesterol	2 mg
Sodium	245 mg
Fiber	3 g

Greek salad

Serves: 8

Preheat to 450 F. Lightly coat a baking sheet with cooking spray.

To make the vinaigrette, whisk together the vinegar, lemon juice, oregano, salt and pepper. While whisking, slowly add the olive oil in a thin stream until emulsified. Set aside.

Spread the eggplant cubes in a single layer on the prepared baking sheet. Spray the eggplant with olive oil cooking spray. Roast for 10 minutes. Turn the cubes and roast until softened and lightly golden, 8-10 minutes longer. Set aside and let cool completely.

In a large bowl, combine the spinach, cucumber, tomato, onion and cooled eggplant. Pour the vinaigrette over the salad and toss to mix well and coat evenly. Divide the salad among individual plates. Sprinkle with the olives and feta cheese.

Quick and easy Greek salad — Serves 2

4 c. red- and green-leaf lettuce
½ c. diced cucumber
½ c. diced bell pepper
½ c. diced carrots
½ c. crumbled feta cheese
2 slices red onion
4 pitted olives
4 pepperoncini peppers

Divide the lettuce between two plates. Combine the cucumber, sweet pepper and carrots. Place half of the mixture on each plate. Top with ¼ c. of feta cheese. Slice red onions into ⅛-in. slices. Separate the slices into rings and place on each salad. Garnish with pitted olives and pepperoncini peppers. Drizzle 1 tbsp. of balsamic vinegar dressing on each salad.

Daily servings: *Vegetables* ● ●, *P/D*, ● *Fat* ●

Day 5 menu

Breakfast

½ whole-grain bagel or
1 slice whole-grain toast
Carbohydrates ●

1½ tbsp. jam

1 large grapefruit or
½ small honeydew melon
Fruit ● ●

Calorie-free beverage

Lunch

1 c. canned lentil soup *P/D* ●

6 whole-grain crackers or 1 small
whole-grain roll *Carbohydrates* ●

½ c. raw baby carrots
Vegetables ●

1 c. grapes *Fruit* ●

Calorie-free beverage

Snack

7 smoky almonds *Fat* ●

Dinner

1 serving seared salmon with
salsa *Vegetables* ● , *P/D* ● ● , *Fat* ●

⅔ c. cooked brown rice
Carbohydrates ● ●

Mixed green salad *Vegetables* ● ●

*Combine 2 c. spring mix greens with ½
sliced tomato, ½ sliced cucumber and
red onion.*

2 tbsp. reduced-calorie French
dressing *Fat* ●

Calorie-free beverage

Daily recommended servings

Vegetables (no limit) ● ● ● ●   Fruits (no limit) ● ● ●
Carbohydrates ● ● ● ●   Protein & Dairy (P/D) ● ● ●   Fats ● ● ●

Dietitian's tips

Fish is an important part of a
healthy diet and it's generally
recommended that you eat fish
twice a week.

Seasonings you can use with fish

- Bay (seafood) seasoning
- Cajun (blackening) spice
- Dill
- Italian seasoning
- Garlic-herb blend
- Lemon pepper
- Lemon-dill seasoning
- Paprika and onion
- Smoke (Place fillets onto
  untreated cedar, applewood
  or maple planks, or use similar
  wood chips, and grill.)
- Teriyaki or soy sauce

Marinades you can use with fish

Mix the ingredients from one of
the bullet points in the list below.
Place the mixture along with the
fish fillets in a covered dish or
plastic bag and marinate for
about 30 minutes in the refrigerator (turning the fillets once).

- 1 tsp. olive oil, 2 green onions
  including chopped green tops,
  ¼ c. rice wine vinegar
- ¼ c. soy sauce, ¼ c. rice wine
  vinegar, 1 tbsp. ginger
  (chopped)
- 1 tsp. olive oil, juice from
  1 lemon, ½ tsp. dried basil,
  2 cloves garlic (chopped)
- ½ c. orange juice, 1 tbsp. Dijon
  mustard, ¼ tsp. black pepper
- ¼ c. orange juice, ¼ c. teriyaki or
  soy sauce, ½ tbsp. garlic
  (chopped)

Flavorful companions for fish

In a covered baking dish, bake
fish at 325 F, topped with one of
the following:

- 4 green onions (chopped),
  lemon slices and ½ c. chicken
  broth
- 1 bay leaf (broken into pieces),
  3 sprigs fresh parsley
  (chopped), ½ c. chicken broth
- 1 tomato (sliced), ¼ tsp.
  oregano, ¼ tsp. basil, black pepper, ½ c. chicken broth
- 1 stalk celery, ¼ c. lemon
  juice, 1 tsp. dill, ½ c.
  chicken broth

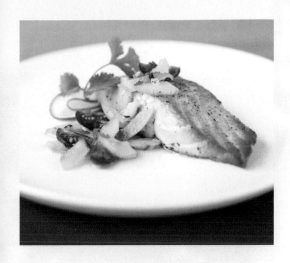

Ingredients list

½ cucumber, peeled, halved lengthwise, seeded, halved lengthwise again, and thinly sliced crosswise

1 c. (6 oz.) cherry tomatoes, quartered

½ yellow or orange bell pepper, seeded and cut into small wedges

2 tbsp. chopped shallot or red onion

1 tbsp. chopped fresh cilantro, plus sprigs for garnish

1 tbsp. fresh lime juice

1½ tsp. canola oil

1 tsp. honey

½ tsp. red pepper flakes

1 tsp. salt

4 salmon fillets, each 5 oz. and about 1 inch thick

¼ tsp. freshly ground black pepper

lime wedges for garnish

Per serving

Calories	243
Protein	29 g
Carbohydrates	6 g
Total fat	11 g
Saturated fat	2 g
Monounsaturated fat	4 g
Cholesterol	78 mg
Sodium	654 mg
Fiber	1 g

Seared salmon with salsa

Serves: 4

In a bowl, combine the cucumber, tomatoes, bell pepper, shallot and chopped cilantro. Toss gently to mix. In a small bowl, whisk together the lime juice, 1 tsp. of the canola oil, the honey, the red pepper flakes and ½ tsp. of the salt. Pour the lime juice mixture over the cucumber mixture and toss gently. Set aside.

Sprinkle the salmon fillets on both sides with the remaining ½ tsp. salt and the black pepper. In a large, nonstick frying pan, heat the remaining ½ tsp. canola oil over medium-high heat. Add the fish to the pan and cook, turning once, until opaque throughout when tested with the tip of a knife, 4-5 minutes on each side.

Transfer the salmon fillets to individual plates and top each with ¼ of the salsa. Garnish the plates with the cilantro sprigs and lime wedges.

Day 6 menu

Breakfast

1 small muffin *Carbohydrates* ●

1 tsp. margarine *Fat* ●

1 tbsp. honey

1 c. berries *Fruit* ●

Calorie-free beverage

Snack

1 serving favorite fruit *Fruit* ●

Lunch

Open-faced ham sandwich *P/D* ●, *Carbohydrates* ●, *Vegetables* ●

Top 1 slice whole-grain bread with 2 oz. lean ham, lettuce leaves, tomato slices and Dijon mustard.

1 c. sliced cucumber or favorite vegetable *Vegetables* ●

2 tbsp. reduced-calorie ranch dressing *Fat* ●

1 small apple *Fruit* ●

Calorie-free beverage

Dinner

Chicken kebabs *P/D* ●, *Vegetables* ● ●, *Fat* ●

Place on skewers 2½ oz. cubed boneless, skinless chicken marinated in fat-free Italian salad dressing and a total of 2 c. of diced mushrooms, green pepper and onion chunks, and cherry tomatoes. Broil or grill.

⅓ c. brown rice with chopped green onions *Carbohydrates* ●

1 serving chocolate pudding pie *P/D* ●, *Carbohydrates* ●

Calorie-free beverage

Daily recommended servings

Vegetables (no limit) ● ● ● ●   Fruits (no limit) ● ● ●
Carbohydrates ● ● ●   Protein & Dairy (P/D) ● ● ●   Fats ● ● ●

Dietitian's tips

Dishes prepared with boneless, skinless chicken are a common staple of a healthy diet. Here are simple ways to vary your menu.

Seasonings you can use with chicken

*   Barbecue sauce
*   Chili sauce
*   Curry powder, salt and pepper
*   Dijon-style mustard and honey (equal parts)
*   Italian seasoning
*   Lemon-herb blend
*   Pineapple (crushed) and onion (chopped)
*   Smoke (Plank the chicken onto untreated hickory, applewood or maple planks, or use wood chips, and grill.)

*   Tarragon and lemon juice
*   Teriyaki or soy sauce

Marinades to use with chicken

Mix the ingredients from one of the bullet points below. Place the chicken in the mixture and marinate for about 1 hour (turning the chicken once).

*   1 tsp. olive oil, 2 cloves garlic (chopped), Cajun seasoning, ¼ c. lemon juice
*   1 tsp. olive oil, juice from 1 lemon and 1 lime, 1 tsp. ground coriander
*   ¼ c. soy sauce, ¼ c. rice wine vinegar, 1 tbsp. ginger (chopped)
*   ¼ c. lemon juice, ¼ c. apple juice, 1 tbsp. dried onion flakes, 1 tsp. dried basil

Aromatic companions for chicken

In a covered dish, bake skinless chicken at 325 F topped with the ingredients from one of the bullets in the following list:

*   4 tbsp. fresh tarragon (chopped), 4 green onions (chopped), 1 c. chicken broth
*   2 dried apricots (chopped), ½ onion (chopped), 1 tbsp. thyme, ¼ c. chicken broth
*   1 apple (peeled and chopped), ½ tsp. sage, 1 c. chicken broth

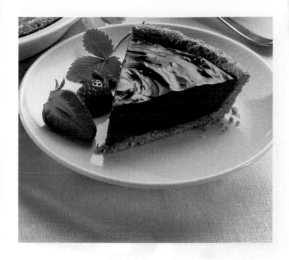

Ingredients list

Crust

8 whole graham crackers
⅔ c. 100 percent unprocessed
    wheat bran
2 tbsp. sugar
¼ tsp. ground cinnamon
2 egg whites

Filling

⅓ c. cornstarch
⅓ c. sugar
⅓ c. unsweetened cocoa powder
3½ c. fat-free milk
2 tsp. vanilla extract
16 strawberries, hulled

Per serving

Calories	191
Protein	7 g
Carbohydrates	38 g
Total fat	2 g
Saturated fat	<1 g
Monounsaturated fat	0 g
Cholesterol	2 mg
Sodium	156 mg
Fiber	4 g

Chocolate pudding pie

Serves: 8

Preheat the oven to 350 F. Coat a 9-inch pie pan with nonstick cooking spray.

To make the crust, in a food processor, process the graham crackers and wheat bran to fine crumbs. Add the sugar, cinnamon and egg whites and process until all the crumbs are dampened. Put the mixture in the prepared pan and firmly pat and press it over the bottom and sides of the pan, taking care not to make the edges too thick.

Bake until crust is lightly browned, feels firm and gives to moderate pressure, about 15 minutes. If overbaked, it will be brittle when cold. Cool completely, about 1 hour.

To make the filling, into a heavy saucepan, sift together the cornstarch, sugar and cocoa powder. Gradually whisk in the milk. Place over medium heat and cook, whisking constantly, until the mixture thickens and boils, about 7 minutes. Reduce heat to medium low and boil gently, whisking constantly, 2 minutes longer. Remove from heat and press a piece of plastic wrap directly onto the surface of the mixture to prevent a skin from forming. Cool 30 minutes.

Remove the plastic from the filling and stir in the vanilla. Pour the filling into the crust and refrigerate until set, at least 2 hours.

Cut into wedges to serve and garnish with strawberries.

Day 7 menu

Breakfast

1 pancake *Carbohydrates ●, Fat ●, Fruit ●*

Top a 4-inch-diameter pancake with ¾ c. berries, 1 tsp. margarine and 1½ tbsp. syrup.

1 c. skim milk *P/D ●*

Calorie-free beverage

Snack

10 baked tortilla chips *Carbohydrates ●*

¼ c. salsa *Vegetables ●*

Lunch

Spinach fruit salad *Vegetables ● ●, Fruit ●*

Top 2 c. baby spinach with ½ c. green pepper strips and water chestnuts and ½ c. mandarin orange sections.

2 tbsp. low-calorie French dressing *Fat ●*

6 whole-grain crackers *Carbohydrates ●*

Calorie-free beverage

Dinner

1 serving Jamaican barbecued pork tenderloin *P/D ● ●*

1 serving warm potato salad (see page 118) *Carbohydrates ●, Fat ●*

6 steamed asparagus spears *Vegetables ●*

½ c. mandarin orange sections or 2 pineapple rings *Fruit ●*

Calorie-free beverage

Daily recommended servings

Vegetables (no limit) ● ● ● ●
Carbohydrates ● ● ● ●
Fruits (no limit) ● ● ●
Protein & Dairy (P/D) ● ● ●
Fats ● ● ●

Dietitian's tips

- When in a pinch, frozen pancakes or waffles may be substituted for homemade. Check the label for calorie content and serving size.
- Frozen berries (strawberries, raspberries, blueberries) can be used in place of fresh berries. However, don't expect the same appearance and texture.
- Salsa is the Spanish word for "sauce." Salsas can be mild, fruity or scorching, smooth or chunky. Salsa isn't only for chips. Try it on potatoes, vegetables, and as a topping for fish, chicken or meats.
- To ease the preparation time for Jamaican barbecued pork tenderloin, you can combine all of the dry spices earlier in the day or even the day before. Store the spice mixture in an airtight container. When it's time to prepare the meal, rub the spice mixture on the pork tenderloin.
- Marinades are seasoned liquids used to add flavor and to tenderize foods. Because most contain an acidic ingredient (juice, vinegar, wine), it's important to not marinate foods too long. The acid can break down the food and make it mushy. Most vegetables and fish require shorter amounts of marinade time — 30 minutes to an hour — whereas large cuts of meat can be marinated up to eight hours.

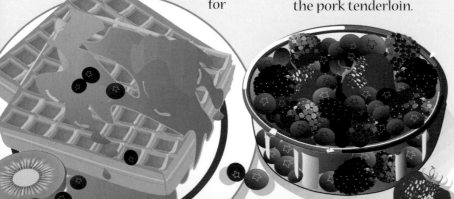

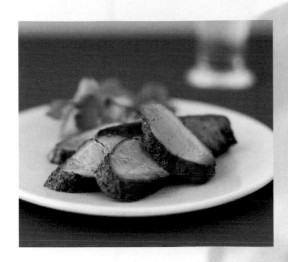

Ingredients list

2 tsp. firmly packed brown sugar
1 tsp. ground allspice
1 tsp. ground cinnamon
½ tsp. ground ginger
½ tsp. onion powder
½ tsp. garlic powder
¼ tsp. cayenne pepper
⅛ tsp. ground cloves
¾ tsp. salt
½ tsp. freshly ground black
    pepper
1 pork tenderloin, about 1 lb.,
    trimmed of visible fat
2 tsp. white vinegar
1½ tsp. dark honey
1 tsp. tomato paste

Per serving

Calories	180
Protein	24 g
Carbohydrates	6 g
Total fat	6 g
Saturated fat	2 g
Monounsaturated fat	3 g
Cholesterol	75 mg
Sodium	508 mg
Fiber	1 g

Jamaican barbecued pork tenderloin

Serves: 4

In a small bowl, combine the brown sugar, allspice, cinnamon, ginger, onion powder, garlic powder, cayenne, cloves, ½ tsp. of the salt and the black pepper. Rub the spice mixture over the pork and let stand for 15 minutes.

In another small bowl, combine the vinegar, honey, tomato paste and the remaining ¼ tsp. salt. Whisk to blend. Set aside.

Prepare a hot fire in a charcoal grill or preheat a gas grill or broiler to medium high or 400 F. Away from the heat source, lightly coat the grill rack or broiler pan with cooking spray. Position the cooking rack 4-6 inches from the heat source.

Place the pork on the grill rack or broiler pan. Grill or broil at medium-high heat, turning several times, until browned on all sides, 3-4 minutes total. Remove to a cooler part of the grill or reduce the heat and continue cooking for 14-16 minutes. Baste with the glaze and continue cooking until the pork is slightly pink inside and a thermometer inserted into the thickest part reads 160 F, 3-4 minutes longer. Transfer to a cutting board and let rest for 5 minutes before slicing.

To serve, slice the pork tenderloin crosswise into pieces and arrange on a warmed serving platter, or divide the slices among individual plates.

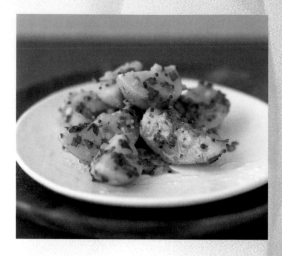

Ingredients list

1 lb. small red or white new
   potatoes (about 1½ inches in
   diameter)
1 tbsp. Dijon mustard
1 tbsp. whole-grain mustard
2 tbsp. rice vinegar
2 tsp. red wine vinegar or sherry
   vinegar
2 tbsp. minced shallot
4 tsp. extra-virgin olive oil
2 tbsp. chopped fresh parsley
¼ tsp. salt
¼ tsp. freshly ground pepper

Per serving

Calories	89
Protein	3 g
Carbohydrates	15 g
Total fat	3 g
Saturated fat	0 g
Monounsaturated fat	2 g
Cholesterol	0 mg
Sodium	202 mg
Fiber	2 g

Warm potato salad

Serves: 6

Put the potatoes in a saucepan, add water to cover, and bring to a boil over high heat. Reduce the heat to medium and cook, uncovered, until the potatoes are tender, 15-20 minutes. Drain and let stand until just cool enough to handle. Cut each potato in half (or quarters, if the potatoes are large) and place in a warmed serving dish.

In a small bowl, whisk together the mustards, the vinegars, and the shallot until well blended. While whisking, slowly drizzle in the olive oil to make a thick dressing. Stir in the parsley, salt and pepper. Pour the dressing over the warm potatoes, mix gently, and serve.

Vegetables

(25 calories in a serving)

Best foods	Amount in 1 serving	Good foods	Amount in 1 serving
Artichoke	$\frac{1}{2}$ bud	Canned vegetables	$\frac{1}{2}$ cup
Asparagus	$\frac{1}{2}$ cup or 6 spears	Marinara sauce	$\frac{1}{4}$ cup
Bamboo shoots	$\frac{1}{2}$ cup	Pickle, sour	1 large
Bean sprouts	1 cup	Pizza sauce	$\frac{1}{4}$ cup
Beets	$\frac{1}{2}$ cup sliced	Salsa	$\frac{1}{4}$ cup
Bell pepper	1 medium	Sauerkraut	$\frac{2}{3}$ cup
Broccoflower	1 cup	Soup	
Broccoli	1 cup florets or spears	• Broth-based	1 cup
Brussels sprouts	4 sprouts	• Tomato	$\frac{1}{3}$ cup
Cabbage, cooked	1 cup	• Vegetable	$\frac{1}{3}$ cup
Cabbage, raw	1 $\frac{1}{2}$ cups	Tomato paste	$\frac{1}{4}$ cup
Carrots	1 or $\frac{1}{2}$ cup baby	Tomato sauce	$\frac{1}{8}$ cup
Cauliflower	1 cup florets	Vegetable juice	$\frac{1}{2}$ cup
Celery	4 medium stalks		
Cherry tomatoes	8 or about 1 cup		
Cucumber	1 or 1 cup sliced		
Eggplant, cooked	1 cup pieces		
Green beans	$\frac{3}{4}$ cup		
Green onions	$\frac{3}{4}$ cup		
Kale, cooked	$\frac{2}{3}$ cup		
Lettuce	2 cups shredded		
Mushrooms	1 cup whole		
Okra	$\frac{1}{2}$ cup		
Onions	$\frac{1}{2}$ cup sliced		
Peas, green	$\frac{1}{4}$ cup		
Radishes	10 small		
Scallions	3		
Spinach, cooked	$\frac{1}{2}$ cup		
Spinach, raw	2 cups		
Squash, summer	$\frac{3}{4}$ cup sliced		
Tomatillo	$\frac{1}{2}$ cup diced		
Tomato	1 medium		
Water chestnuts	$\frac{3}{4}$ cup		
Zucchini	$\frac{3}{4}$ cup		

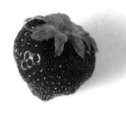

Fruits

(60 calories in a serving)

Best foods	Amount in 1 serving	Good foods	Amount in 1 serving
Apple	1 small	Apple juice	$1/2$ cup
Apricots	4 whole	Applesauce, unsweetened	$1/2$ cup
Banana	1 small or $1/2$ large		
Berries, mixed	1 cup	Cranberry juice	$1/2$ cup
Blackberries	$1/2$ cup	Cranberry juice, reduced-calorie	1 cup
Blueberries	$3/4$ cup		
Cantaloupe	1 cup cubed	Dates	3
Cantaloupe wedge	$1/4$ small melon	Figs, dried	3 small
Cherries	1 cup or about 1 dozen	Grapefruit juice	$1/2$ cup
Figs, fresh	2 small	Juice bar, frozen	3-ounce bar
Grapefruit	1 small or $1/2$ large	Orange juice	$1/2$ cup
Grapes	1 cup	Pineapple juice	$1/2$ cup
Honeydew melon	1 cup cubed	Prunes	3
Kiwi	1 large	Raisins	2 tablespoons
Mandarin oranges	$1/2$ cup sections		
Mango	$1/2$ cup diced		
Melon balls	7		
Mixed fruit	$1/2$ cup		
Nectarine	1		
Orange	1 medium		
Papaya	$1/3$ medium		
Peach	1 large		
Pear	1 small		
Pineapple	$1/2$ cup cubed or 2 rings		
Plums	2		
Raspberries	1 cup		
Strawberries	$1 1/2$ cups whole		
Tangerine	1 large or $3/4$ cup		
Watermelon	$1 1/4$ cups cubed or small wedge		

Carbohydrates

(70 calories in a serving)

Best foods	Amount in 1 serving	Good foods	Amount in 1 serving
Bagel, whole-grain	1/2	Animal crackers	6
Barley, cooked	1/3 cup	Baked chips, low-fat	10 chips
Bread, sourdough	1 slice	Breadsticks, crispy	1, 6- to 8-inch
Bread, whole-grain	1 slice	Corn	1/2 cup
Bulgur, cooked	1/2 cup	Corn on the cob	1/2 large ear
Cereal, whole-grain	1/2 cup	Corn tortillas	1
English muffin, whole-grain	1/2	Crackers	
Grits, uncooked	2 tablespoons	• Cheese	14 small
Kasha, (buckwheat groats, cooked)	1/2 cup	• Snack	20 bite size, 5 round
Oatmeal, cooked	1/2 cup	• Triple-rye	1
Pasta, whole-grain, cooked	1/2 cup	• Wheat	6
Pita bread, whole-grain	1/2 circle, 6-inch diameter	Melba rounds	6
Pumpkin, cooked	1 1/2 cups	Muffin, any flavor	1 small
Rice, brown, cooked	1/3 cup	Orzo, cooked	1/4 cup
Roll, whole-grain	1 small	Pancake	1, 4-inch diameter
Rutabaga, cooked	3/4 cup	Popcorn, microwave, low-fat	2 cups
Shredded wheat	1 biscuit or 1/2 cup spoon-sized	Potato	
Squash, winter, cooked	1 cup	• Baby	3
Sweet potato, baked	1/2 large	• Baked	1/2 medium
Turnips, cooked	1/3 cup	• Mashed	1/2 cup
		Pretzels, sticks	30
		Pretzels, twists	3
		Rice, white, cooked	1/2 cup
		Rice or popcorn cakes	3
		Sorbet	1/3 cup
		Soup, chicken noodle	1 cup
		Waffle	1, 4-inch square

Protein/Dairy

(110 calories in a serving)

Best foods	Amount in 1 serving	Good foods	Amount in 1 serving
Beans	1/2 cup	Beef, lean	1 1/2 ounces
Chicken	2 1/2 ounces	Cheese	
Clams, canned	1/2 cup	• Cheddar, low-fat	2 ounces
Cod	3 ounces	• Colby, low-fat	2 ounces
Crab	3 ounces	• Cottage, low-fat	2/3 cup
Egg whites	4	• Feta	1/4 cup
Fish	3 ounces	• Mozzarella, part-skim	1/3 cup shredded
Garbanzos	1/3 cup	• Parmesan, grated	4 tablespoons
Halibut	3 ounces	• Ricotta, part-skim	1/4 cup
Lentils	1/2 cup	• Swiss, low-fat	2 ounces
Milk, skim or 1 percent	1 cup	Duck, breast	3 ounces
Peas	3/4 cup	Egg	1 medium
Pheasant	3 ounces	Egg substitute	1/2 cup
Salmon	3 ounces	Frozen yogurt, fat-free	1/2 cup
Shrimp	3 ounces	Ice cream, fat-free, vanilla	1/2 cup
Soybeans, green (edamame)	1/2 cup	Lamb, lean cuts with no fat	2 ounces
Tofu	1/2 cup	Milk, 2 percent	1 cup
Tuna, canned in water	3 ounces or 1/2 cup	Pork, lean cuts with no fat	2 ounces
Turkey	3 ounces	Veal	2 ounces
Vegetarian burger, black bean	3-ounce pattie	Yogurt, fat-free, reduced-calorie	1 cup
Venison	3 ounces		

Fats and Sweets

(Fats 45 calories in a serving · Sweets 75 calories in a serving)

Best fats	Amount in 1 serving
Avocado	$^1/_6$
Nuts	
• Almonds	7 whole
• Cashews	4 whole
• Peanuts	8 whole
• Pecans	4 halves
• Walnuts	4 halves
Oil	
• Canola	1 teaspoon
• Olive	1 teaspoon
Olives	9 large
Peanut butter	$1^1/_2$ teaspoons
Seeds	
• Sesame	1 tablespoon
• Sunflower	1 tablespoon

Sweets	Amount in 1 serving
Angel food cake	1 small slice
Fruit spread	$1^1/_2$ tablespoons
Gelatin dessert	$^1/_2$ cup
Honey	1 tablespoon
Jam	$1^1/_2$ tablespoons
Maple syrup	$1^1/_2$ tablespoons

Good fats	Amount in 1 serving
Butter, regular	1 teaspoon
Cream	
• Half-and-half	2 tablespoons
• Sour	$1^1/_2$ tablespoons
• Sour, fat-free	3 tablespoons
• Heavy (whipping)	1 tablespoon liquid or 4 tablespoons whipped
• Nondairy topping	$^1/_2$ cup
Cream cheese	
• Fat-free	3 tablespoons
• Regular	1 tablespoon
Margarine	
• Regular	1 teaspoon
Mayonnaise	
• Fat-free	4 tablespoon
• Reduced-calorie	1 tablespoon
• Regular	2 teaspoons
Salad dressing	
• Low-calorie	2 tablespoons
• Regular	2 teaspoons
Tartar sauce	1 tablespoon

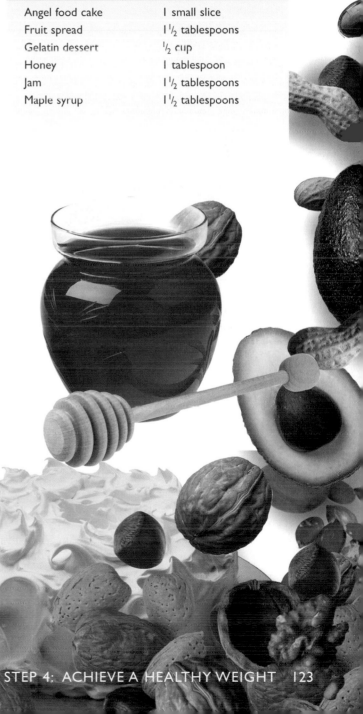

Additional recipes!

Soft taco with Southwestern vegetables

Ingredients list

1 tbsp. olive oil
1 medium red onion, chopped
1 c. diced yellow summer squash
1 c. diced green zucchini
3 large garlic cloves, minced
4 medium tomatoes, seeded and
  chopped
1 jalapeno pepper, seeded and
  chopped
1 c. corn, frozen
½ c. fresh cilantro, chopped
1 c. canned pinto or black beans,
  rinsed
4 8-in. fat-free tortillas
½ c. salsa

Per serving

Calories	295
Protein	10 g
Carbohydrates	55 g
Total fat	6 g
Saturated fat	1 g
Monounsaturated fat	3 g
Cholesterol	0 mg
Sodium	221 mg
Fiber	10 g

Serves: 4

Heat oil in large skillet; add onion and cook until tender. Add squash and zucchini, stir and continue cooking about 5 minutes. Add garlic, ½ of the tomatoes and all of the pepper. Reduce heat to medium-low and cook until flavorful. Add corn and stir and cook until kernels are tender-crisp. Add the cilantro, the remaining tomatoes and beans. Stir together and remove from heat.

Warm the tortillas on a hot, dry skillet. Fill each with the vegetable mixture. Top with salsa and serve.

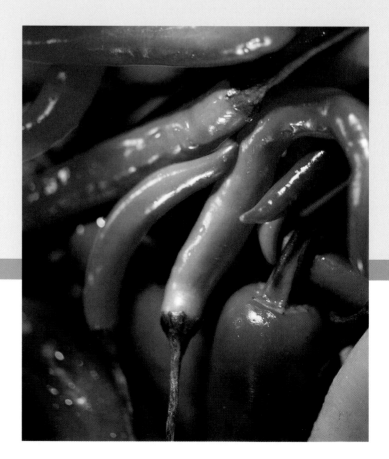

Pyramid servings

Vegetables	2
Fruits	
Carbohydrates	2
Protein & Dairy	1
Fats	

Green beans with red pepper and garlic

Ingredients list

1 lb. green beans, stems trimmed
2 tsp. olive oil
1 red bell pepper, seeded and cut
1 tsp. chile paste or red pepper
   flakes
1 clove garlic, finely chopped
1 tsp. sesame oil
½ tsp. salt
¼ tsp. freshly ground black pepper

Per serving

Calories	50
Protein	2 g
Carbohydrates	7 g
Total fat	2 g
Saturated fat	1 g
Monounsaturated fat	1 g
Cholesterol	0 mg
Sodium	201 mg
Fiber	3 g

Pyramid servings

Vegetables	2
Fruits	
Carbohydrates	
Protein & Dairy	
Fats	

Serves: 6

Green beans, also known as string beans or snap beans, are available year-round. To preserve their fresh flavor and texture, parboil the beans, immerse them in ice water to set their color, and then sauté briefly.

Cut the beans into 2-inch pieces. Bring a large saucepan ¾ full of water to a boil. Add the beans and cook until they turn bright green and are tender-crisp, about 1 to 3 minutes. Drain the beans, then plunge them into a bowl of ice water to stop the cooking. Drain again and set aside.

In a large frying pan, heat the olive oil over medium heat. Add the bell pepper and toss and stir for about 1 minute. Add the beans and sauté for 1 minute longer. Add the chile paste and garlic and toss and stir for one minute longer. The beans will be tender and bright green. Drizzle with the sesame oil and season with the salt and black pepper.

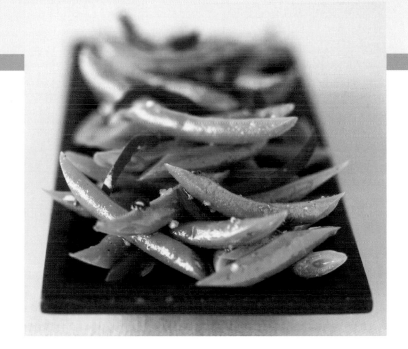

Ingredients list

2 tbsp. plus 2 tsp. olive oil
1½ tbsp. all-purpose (plain) flour
2 cloves garlic, minced
1 c. (8 fl. oz.) plain soy (soya) milk
1 c. (8 fl. oz.) vegetable or chicken stock
2 green onions, including tender tops, sliced
½ c. (4 oz.) dry-packed sun-dried tomatoes, soaked in water to rehydrate, drained, and chopped
10 oz. fresh cremini or shiitake mushrooms, sliced
1 shallot, minced
1 tbsp. chopped fresh flat-leaf (Italian) parsley
¼ tsp. salt
6 c. (12 oz.) baby spinach leaves, chopped
2 c. (16 oz.) fat-free ricotta cheese
¾ c. (3 oz.) grated Parmesan cheese
1 egg white
12 no-boil spinach lasagna sheets, about 7 by 3½ in.
1 tbsp. chopped fresh basil

Per serving

Calories	288
Protein	17 g
Carbohydrates	39 g
Total fat	8 g
Saturated fat	2 g
Monounsaturated fat	4 g
Cholesterol	6 mg
Sodium	526 mg
Fiber	4 g

Serves: 8

In a saucepan, heat the 2 tbsp. olive oil over medium-high heat. Whisk in the flour and cook for 1 to 2 minutes, stirring constantly. Add the garlic and continue to whisk until the garlic is fragrant, about 30 seconds. Whisk in the soy milk and stock all at once. Cook and stir until slightly thickened. Remove from the heat and stir in the green onions and sun-dried tomatoes. Set the sauce aside.

In a large nonstick frying pan, heat 1 tsp. of the olive oil over medium-high heat. Add the mushrooms and shallot and sauté until lightly browned, about 10 minutes. Stir in the parsley and salt. Transfer to a bowl and set aside to cool.

In the same pan, heat the remaining 1 tsp. olive oil over medium-high heat. Add the spinach and stir quickly until the spinach is wilted but still bright green. Remove from the heat. Let cool slightly.

In a large bowl, beat together the ricotta, ½ c. (2 oz.) of the Parmesan, and the egg white. Stir in the spinach and set aside.

Preheat the oven to 375 F. Lightly coat a 9-by-13-in. baking dish with cooking spray. Spread ½ c. (4 fl. oz.) of the sauce in the dish and cover with 3 sheets of the pasta. Spoon half of the spinach mixture onto the pasta and spread gently. Cover with 3 more pasta sheets. Top with another ½ c. of sauce. Spread the mushroom mixture on top and cover with another ½ c. of sauce, then another layer of pasta. Spoon in the remaining spinach filling and top with the last 3 pasta sheets. Add the remaining sauce and the remaining ¼ c. (1 oz.) Parmesan. Cover with foil and bake for 25 minutes. Remove the foil and bake until golden, about 10 minutes longer. Let stand for 10 minutes before serving. Garnish with the basil.

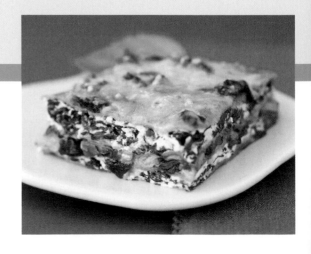

Pyramid servings

Vegetables	3
Fruits	
Carbohydrates	1
Protein & Dairy	1
Fats	1

Grilled pineapple

Ingredients list

Marinade
2 tbsp. dark honey
1 tbsp. olive oil
1 tbsp. fresh lime juice
1 tsp. ground cinnamon
¼ tsp. ground cloves

1 firm yet ripe pineapple
8 wooden skewers, soaked in water
    for 30 minutes, or metal skewers
1 tbsp. dark rum (optional)
1 tbsp. grated lime zest

Per serving

Calories	79
Protein	1 g
Carbohydrates	15 g
Total fat	2 g
Saturated fat	1 g
Monounsaturated fat	1 g
Cholesterol	0 mg
Sodium	1 mg
Fiber	1 g

Pyramid servings

Vegetables	
Fruits	1
Carbohydrates	
Protein & Dairy	
Fats	

Serves: 8

Prepare a hot fire in a charcoal grill or preheat a gas grill or broiler (grill). Away from the heat source, lightly coat the grill rack or broiler pan with cooking spray. Position the cooking rack 4-6 inches from the heat source.

To make the marinade, in a small bowl, combine the honey, olive oil, lime juice, cinnamon and cloves and whisk to blend. Set aside.

Cut off the crown of leaves and the base of the pineapple. Stand the pineapple upright and, using a large, sharp knife, pare off the skin, cutting downward just below the surface in long, vertical strips and leaving the small brown "eyes" on the fruit. Lay the pineapple on its side. Aligning the knife blade with the diagonal rows of eyes, cut a shallow furrow, following a spiral pattern around the pineapple, to remove all the eyes. Stand the peeled pineapple upright and cut it in half lengthwise. Place each pineapple half cut-side down and cut it lengthwise into 4 long wedges; slice away the core. Cut each wedge crosswise into 3 pieces. Thread the 3 pineapple pieces onto each skewer.

Lightly brush the pineapple with the marinade. Grill or broil, turning once and basting once or twice with the remaining marinade, until tender and golden, about 5 minutes on each side.

Remove the pineapple from the skewers and place on a platter or individual serving plates. Brush with the rum, if using, and sprinkle with the lime zest. Serve hot or warm.

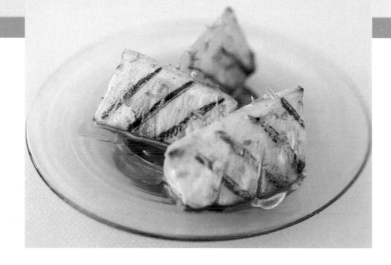

Banana-oatmeal hotcakes with spiced maple syrup

Ingredients list

½ c. (5½ oz.) maple syrup
½ cinnamon stick
3 whole cloves
½ c. (1½ oz.) old-fashioned rolled oats
1 c. (8 fl. oz.) water
2 tbsp. firmly packed light brown sugar
2 tbsp. canola oil
½ c. (2½ oz.) whole-wheat flour
½ c. (2½ oz.) all-purpose flour
1½ tsp. baking powder
¼ tsp. baking soda
¼ tsp. salt
¼ tsp. ground cinnamon
½ c. (4 fl. oz.) 1 percent low-fat milk
¼ c. (2 oz.) fat-free plain yogurt
1 banana, peeled and mashed
1 egg, lightly beaten

Per serving

Calories	268
Protein	6 g
Carbohydrates	48 g
Total fat	6 g
Saturated fat	1 g
Monounsaturated fat	3 g
Cholesterol	36 mg
Sodium	230 mg
Fiber	3 g

Serves: 6

In a small saucepan, combine the maple syrup, cinnamon stick and cloves. Place over medium heat and bring to a boil. Remove from the heat and let steep for 15 minutes. Remove the cinnamon stick and cloves with a slotted spoon. Set the syrup aside and keep warm.

In a large microwave-safe bowl, combine the oats and water. Microwave on high until the oats are creamy and tender, about 3 minutes. Stir in the brown sugar and canola oil. Set aside to cool slightly.

In a bowl, combine the flours, baking powder, baking soda, salt and ground cinnamon. Whisk to blend.

Add the milk, yogurt and mashed banana to the oats and stir until well blended. Beat in the egg. Add the flour mixture to the oat mixture and stir just until moistened.

Place a nonstick frying pan or griddle over medium heat. When a drop of water sizzles as it hits the pan, spoon ¼ c. (2 fl. oz.) pancake batter into the pan. Cook until the top surface of the pancake is covered with bubbles and the edges are lightly browned, about 2 minutes. Turn and cook until the bottom is well browned and the pancake is cooked through, 1 to 2 minutes longer. Repeat with the remaining pancake batter.

Place the pancakes on warmed individual plates. Drizzle with the warm syrup and serve immediately.

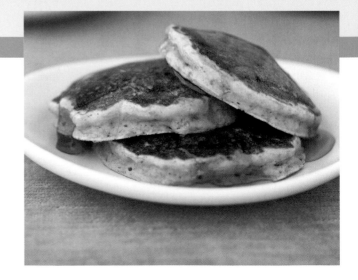

Pyramid servings

Vegetables	
Fruits	1
Carbohydrates	2
Protein & Dairy	
Fats	1

Muesli breakfast bars

Ingredients list

2½ c. (7½ oz.) old-fashioned rolled oats
½ c. (2 oz.) soy flour
½ c. (1½ oz.) fat-free dry milk
½ c. (1½ oz.) toasted wheat germ
½ c. (2 oz.) sliced almonds or chopped pecans, toasted
½ c. (1½ oz.) dried apples, chopped
½ c. (3 oz.) raisins
½ tsp. salt
1 c. (12 oz.) dark honey
½ c. (5 oz.) natural unsalted peanut butter
1 tbsp. olive oil
2 tsp. vanilla extract

Per bar

Calories	162
Protein	5 g
Carbohydrates	25 g
Total fat	5 g
Saturated fat	1 g
Monounsaturated fat	3 g
Cholesterol	1 mg
Sodium	60 mg
Fiber	3 g

Makes: 24 bars

The original breakfast cereal called muesli (a German word meaning "mixture") combined rolled oats with nuts and fruit. The bars here are perfect for breakfast-on-the-go or for a healthy snack anytime.

Preheat the oven to 325 F. Lightly coat a 9-by-13 in. baking pan with olive oil cooking spray.

In a large bowl, combine the oats, flour, dry milk, wheat germ, almonds, apples, raisins and salt. Stir well to blend, and set aside.

In a small saucepan, stir together the honey, peanut butter and olive oil over medium-low heat until well blended. Don't let the mixture boil. Stir in the vanilla. Add the warm honey mixture to the dry ingredients and stir quickly until well combined. The mixture should be sticky but not wet.

Pat the mixture evenly into the prepared baking pan. Press firmly to remove any air pockets. Bake just until the edges begin to brown, about 25 minutes. Let cool in the pan on a wire rack for 10 minutes, then cut into 24 bars. When just cool enough to handle, remove the bars from the pan and place on the rack to cool completely. Store in airtight containers in the refrigerator.

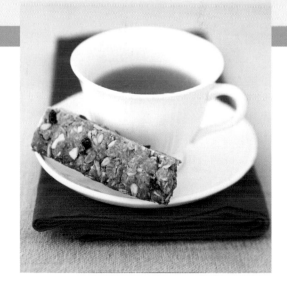

Pyramid servings

Vegetables	
Fruits	1
Carbohydrates	1
Protein & Dairy	
Fats	1

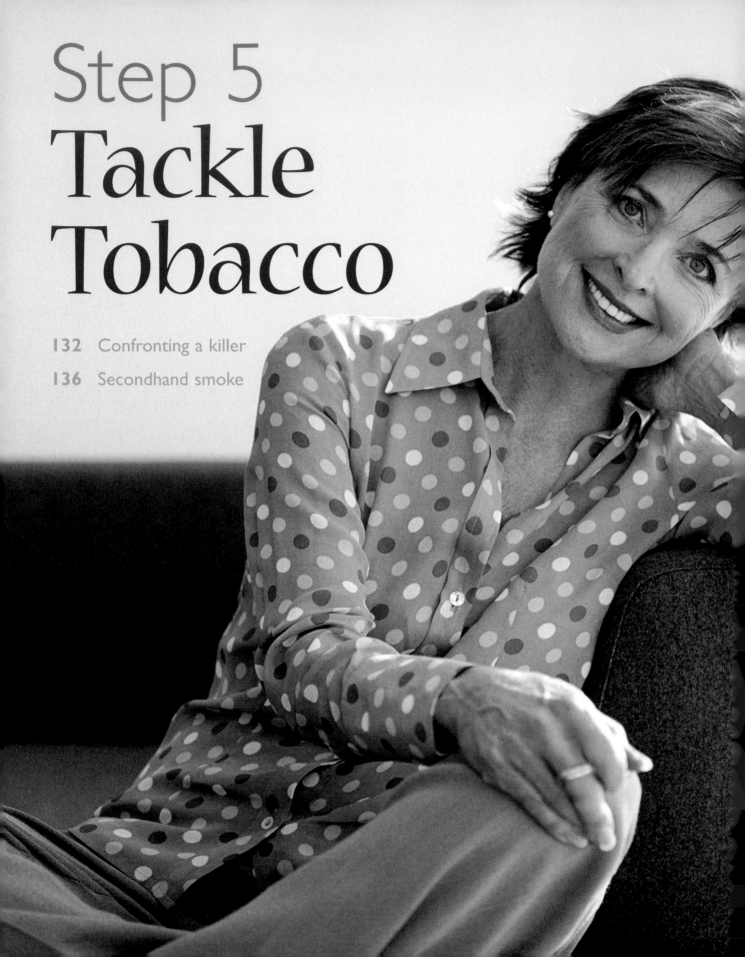

Step 5
Tackle Tobacco

A visit with Dr. Lowell Dale

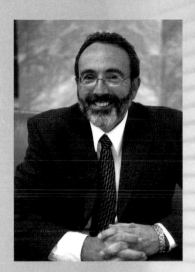

Lowell Dale, M.D.
Nicotine Dependence Center

I think as we look at the impact of smoking on our society — where even now 25 percent of people in the United States smoke — I don't think there's anyone who hasn't been affected. We've all had a loved one, a friend, a relative who's had a smoking-related disease. We also know that secondhand smoke can be very harmful. So I think it's important that, even if you don't smoke, you understand the negative effects of tobacco use and how to eliminate or avoid them.

When it comes to stopping smoking, I like to stress the positive effects of stopping on your health, the health of your family, your relationships and the financial gains involved, rather than the negatives of continued smoking. I stress that not smoking really is important for overall good health. But we as a society also need to recognize that it's difficult to stop and that most people need support. They shouldn't think that they must go it alone when stopping.

We're really just beginning to understand how to treat nicotine dependence with the many medicines we currently have, and we expect that soon there will be several new drugs available. Telephone quitlines are also coming into their own, increasing accessibility to effective counseling services. And we see insurance companies and Medicare providing coverage for counseling services and medications. So there are tremendous opportunities for people to get the assistance they need to really make a stop attempt successful.

Q: Is stopping smoking 'cold turkey' a good idea?

A: Most people who've been successful in stopping smoking have quit "cold turkey," which I define as setting a specific stop date and then sticking to it, with or without the aid of medications. This seems to be much more effective than gradually tapering down on the number of cigarettes smoked each day. Many people who try to taper compensate by inhaling more deeply, or smoking more of each cigarette and thus are not really reducing their exposure to nicotine. They reach a certain number of cigarettes and just aren't able to reduce the amount further. Using one or more of the various medications available for stopping smoking makes the "cold turkey" approach even more likely to succeed. Certainly, combining the two strategies can be effective, too. For example, set your target quit date for one to two weeks in the future, begin a gradual taper of the number of cigarettes you smoke, and then on the quit date stop all cigarettes and use medications and behavioral strategies to stay tobacco-free.

Q: As a nonsmoker, how long do I have to be exposed to secondhand smoke before I suffer ill effects?

A: Many factors influence exposure and risk, including the concentration of secondhand smoke present, the amount of ventilation and the length of exposure. Studies have shown that as little as five minutes of exposure to secondhand smoke results in harmful effects to blood vessels. This suggests that any amount of exposure is too much.

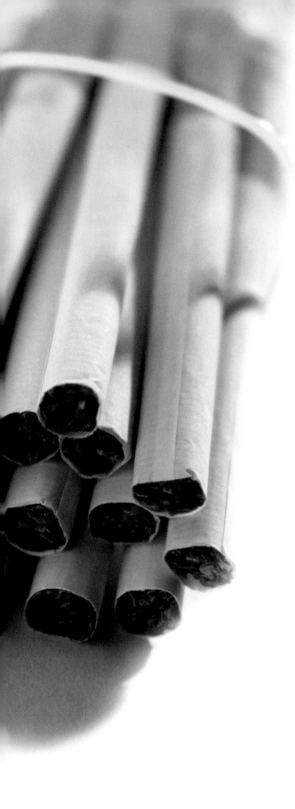

Confronting a killer

Tobacco kills. Individuals who smoke are more likely to develop disease and die earlier than those who don't. It's that simple.

Despite all of the warnings about its dangers, tobacco remains a serious health threat. Approximately 45 million Americans smoke — just over 20 percent of the adult population. One in four high school students also smokes.

Most smokers understand the hazards of tobacco. But what they fail to understand is how hard it is to quit. Nicotine is a highly addictive drug, and quitting smoking can be very difficult. In fact, most people fail in their first attempt. But just because you've failed once — or more than once — doesn't mean you can't succeed and that you shouldn't try again.

Consider your options

Your doctor is a valuable resource as you take steps to quit smoking. Following are some ways that people try to quit smoking. Think about what method would work best for you, and then team up with your doctor to get started.

Cold turkey

Cold turkey is the most frequently used method to stop smoking. It's a sudden break from cigarettes. On a chosen day, you quit smoking completely with little or no reduction beforehand. Stopping smoking isn't something you do on a whim. It requires emotional and physical preparation to withstand the strong desire to smoke. Some form of medication is usually recommended.

Taper down

With the taper-down approach, you gradually reduce the number of cigarettes you smoke until you don't smoke any at all. Medication is generally recommended with this approach, as well.

Individual counseling

Counseling involves working one-on-one with a health care professional who can provide advice and support. This setting allows you to discuss your worries of not being able to stop smoking, and your concerns about weight gain or adjusting to a tobacco-free lifestyle. During counseling sessions, professionals help you gain coping skills, overcome obstacles and learn to live as a nonsmoker. Medication is usually recommended in addition to counseling.

Group support

For some people, the support of a group is critical to quitting smoking. In addition to the aid and encouragement of others trying to give up tobacco, group programs generally offer tools and techniques to help you make it through difficult days. Medication is often one of these tools.

Telephone quitlines

Counseling over the telephone has become an increasingly popular and accessible way for people to receive help for their smoking. Telephone counseling allows participants to receive an intensive intervention that's almost identical to face-to-face consultation, but with greater convenience. To access your state's quitline, try (800) QUIT-NOW or *www.naquitline.org.*

Plan your attack

Success at quitting smoking is a result of planning and commitment, not luck. Develop a plan that addresses how you'll cope with symptoms of nicotine withdrawal, how you'll survive urges to smoke, and how you'll summon family and friends when you need their support. No one plan works for everybody. Develop a strategy that you feel comfortable with and that fits your lifestyle.

Often, stop plans combine several strategies. Studies show that using more than one strategy — such as medication plus counseling — increases your chance of being successful.

The first few days are often the most difficult, but you may continue to experience withdrawal symptoms for several weeks. When the symptoms begin to lessen, you may still have an impulse to smoke at those times you usually would light up, such as after a meal or when driving. You need to plan for these situations, too.

Ask about medication

There are several medications available to help you stop smoking. They help ease withdrawal symptoms and manage cravings. They also allow you to focus on changing behaviors that may have led to your smoking. Remember, though, that medication is only an aid. You still need to be psychologically ready to quit. Medication is only effective among smokers who are motivated to quit.

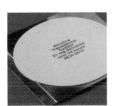

Nicotine patch

A nicotine patch delivers a steady dose of nicotine into your bloodstream through your skin. Most nicotine patch products are available without a prescription. Nicotine patches are used daily for six to 12 weeks and have been shown to be very effective, but they're not a magic cure. The most common side effect is skin irritation that may occur after several weeks of use. If this occurs, after you remove the patch, apply hydrocortisone cream over the area of affected skin. To reduce skin irritation, apply the patch to a different site each day.

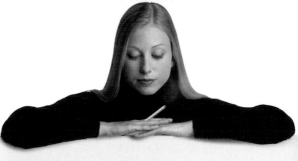

Think you're not in danger — Think again

- Each year, more Americans die of smoking-related diseases than from alcohol, AIDS, drug abuse, car accidents, fire, suicide and murder — combined.

- Smoking is responsible for nearly one in five deaths in the United States. Each year, smoking-related diseases claim about 438,000 American lives.

- On average, smokers die 14 years earlier than do nonsmokers. Smokers between the ages of 35 and 70 have death rates three times higher than do nonsmokers of the same age.

- Smoking accounts for at least 30 percent of all cancer deaths. It's a major risk factor for cancers of the lung, mouth, larynx, pharynx, esophagus, stomach, pancreas, kidney, urinary bladder and cervix.

- Smoking is a major contributor to cardiovascular disease, which includes conditions such as coronary artery disease and stroke. Almost 180,000 Americans die each year of cardiovascular disease — mainly heart attack — caused by smoking.

- Smoking is the No. 1 cause of chronic obstructive pulmonary disease (COPD), which includes emphysema and chronic bronchitis.

Quitters are winners

The benefits of quitting smoking begin almost immediately. If you quit smoking right now, you'll begin to see improvements in your health in just days.

Within 24 hours, the levels of carbon monoxide and nicotine in your circulatory system will decrease significantly. Within a few days of quitting smoking you may breathe easier and your smoker's cough will begin to disappear. You may also notice an improvement in your stamina. Your sense of smell and taste also will improve.

By the end of your first nonsmoking year, your risk of heart attack will decrease by half, and by five years it'll be almost the same as that of individuals who have never smoked.

The American Cancer Society believes that quitting smoking immediately decreases your risk of esophageal or pancreatic cancer. Within seven years, your risk of bladder cancer will drop to that of a nonsmoker. And after 10 to 15 years, your statistical odds of getting cancer of the lung, larynx or mouth will approach that of people who have never smoked.

You CAN DO IT!

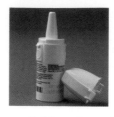

Nicotine nasal spray

Nicotine nasal spray (Nicotrol) delivers nicotine into the bloodstream through the lining of your nose. Among the various nicotine replacement products, it provides the most rapid relief of withdrawal symptoms. The nasal spray is available only with a doctor's prescription. The spray can cause a hot, peppery feeling in your nose, along with coughing and sneezing, watering eyes and throat irritation. These side effects usually improve within the first week of use.

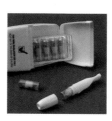

Nicotine inhaler

A nicotine inhaler (Nicotrol) resembles a short cigarette with a plastic mouthpiece. However, the nicotine isn't inhaled. Rather, it's puffed, which allows nicotine to be absorbed into your bloodstream through the lining of your mouth. The nicotine inhaler is available only with a doctor's prescription. You may experience irritation in your mouth or throat. Drink water to relieve any soreness or dryness.

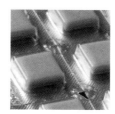

Nicotine gum and lozenges

Nicotine polacrilex is a gum-like resin that delivers nicotine into your bloodstream by way of the lining of your mouth. Bite into a piece of the gum a few times and then park it between your cheek and gum. Nicotine lozenges are made of the same material, but slowly dissolve in your mouth. Periodically move the lozenge from one side of your mouth to the other. The lozenges also deliver nicotine into your bloodstream through the lining of your mouth. The goal with each of these products is to use enough to maintain your nicotine level and hold in check any withdrawal symptoms. Gradually decrease the amounts you use as your desire for cigarettes is reduced. Both products are available in pharmacies without a prescription.

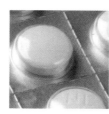

Non-nicotine medication

The medication bupropion (Zyban) doesn't contain nicotine. Bupropion raises the level of the brain chemical dopamine, the same chemical released by nicotine. Bupropion helps reduce the symptoms and discomfort felt when you stop smoking. This medication, taken as a pill, is available only with a doctor's prescription. Side effects include dry mouth, headache, difficulty sleeping, decreased appetite and nausea. To lessen stomach symptoms, bupropion may be taken with food.

Many new medications for treating nicotine addiction and tobacco use are under study. They include both nicotine replacement medications and non-nicotine products.

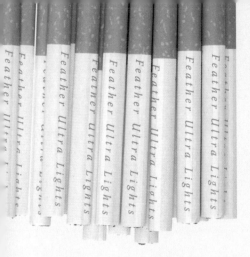

Don't be fooled

Tobacco is tobacco. One form isn't any less dangerous than another. Using other types of tobacco products or cigarette alternatives endangers your health just as much as regular cigarettes.

Light cigarettes

Cigarette companies have implied over the years that so-called light cigarettes — those that are low-tar, low-nicotine — are safer and cause fewer health risks. But features such as tiny ventilation holes in the filters don't reduce your exposure to harmful chemicals in tobacco. And smokers addicted to nicotine will get their fix of nicotine, regardless. They may com-

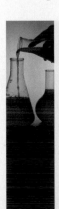

A Mayo Clinic study found that smokeless tobacco raises short-term adrenaline levels in the bloodstream by more than 50 percent and also causes surges in heart rate and blood pressure.

pensate for the diluted smoke by taking more frequent puffs, inhaling more deeply or simply smoking more cigarettes. People who smoke light cigarettes may actually take in more tar and nicotine than they would with regular cigarettes. Switching to low-tar, low-nicotine cigarettes doesn't decrease your risk of lung cancer, emphysema, heart attack or other diseases.

Cigars

Cigar use in the United States is on the rise. Much of the increase can be attributed to adults with higher levels of income and education. Evidence also suggests many cigar users are tobacco newcomers: teenagers and young adult males.

Although cigar smokers often don't fully inhale smoke into their lungs, they're still exposed to smoke in their oral cavity, as well as to the secondhand smoke in the smoking environment.

Considering that cigar smoke contains as many poisonous chemicals as cigarette smoke, cigar smokers are at risk of the same smoking-related illnesses. Cigar smokers and cigarette smokers have similar risk levels of cancers of the mouth, throat and esophagus. And cigar smokers are still four to 10 times more likely to die of cancers of the lung and larynx than are nonsmokers.

Pipes

Studies on the risks of lung or heart disease in people who smoke only a pipe compared with people who smoke only cigarettes or cigars are

limited. However, pipe smoking is associated with cancers of the lip and mouth, and pipe smoking clearly increases the level of carbon monoxide in your blood, putting you at increased risk of cardiovascular and lung disease.

Snuff and chewing tobacco

Similar to cigar use, use of snuff and chewing tobacco is on the rise. Some people have switched to smokeless tobacco to get around the increasing number of smoking bans in restaurants and public places. For years, snuff and chewing tobacco have been thought to be a safe alternative to cigarette smoking, but they're not safe at all.

In addition to long-term nicotine dependence, possible health risks associated with smokeless tobacco include cancers of the mouth, throat, cheek, gums, lip and tongue. Frequently, a white, leathery patch forms at the location in your mouth where the tobacco is held. This condition, called leukoplakia, is a forerunner to cancer.

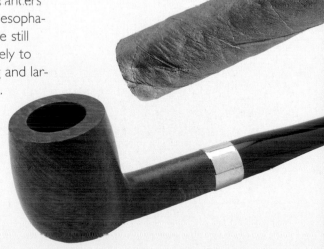

Secondhand smoke

Evidence suggests that the hazards of tobacco are strongest for smokers. But regular exposure to other people's tobacco smoke — secondhand smoke — also may threaten your health. Secondhand smoke may cause or contribute to a number of health conditions from ear infections to cancer.

By avoiding secondhand smoke, you can decrease your risk of getting sick from it.

More than just a gray cloud

Secondhand smoke, also known as passive smoke and environmental tobacco smoke, is a mixture of two types of smoke:

- **Sidestream smoke.** This is smoke that wafts from the burning material.
- **Mainstream smoke.** This is smoke the smoker exhales.

Both types generally contain the same harmful compounds — and a lot of them.

Health experts have long recognized the relationship between secondhand smoke and health risks, and the research exploring their connections is ongoing. Cancer is just one of the known or suspected risks.

Cancer

Secondhand smoke is linked to cancers of the lung, breast, cervix and bladder. Experts believe that secondhand smoke is to blame for roughly 3,000 lung cancer deaths in nonsmokers each year in the United States. Some research indicates that people exposed to a spouse's cigarette smoke for several decades are about 20 percent more likely to have lung cancer. Those who are exposed long-term to secondhand smoke in the workplace or in social settings may increase their lung cancer risk by about 25 percent.

Heart disease

Secondhand smoke is associated with up to 62,000 deaths in the United States each year from heart disease that's caused by narrowing of the blood vessels to the heart.

Childhood illnesses

Secondhand smoke also may have a marked effect on the health of infants and children. Some conditions of concern are:

- **Asthma.** Secondhand smoke may make asthma attacks more frequent and severe in children who already have asthma. Even children without asthma are 40 percent more likely to miss school with a respiratory ailment if they live with at least two smokers. Secondhand smoke is also associated with up to 300,000 cases of bronchitis and pneumonia in infants and toddlers each year.
- **Middle ear conditions.** Children living in households with smokers are more likely to have ear infections or fluid in their ears. Secondhand smoke may be a factor in more than 1 million children's visits to the doctor for middle ear infections every year.
- **Low birth weight and SIDS.** Secondhand smoke is associated with low birth weight. Low birth weight, in turn, has been linked to increased risks of other health problems from childhood into adulthood. Research also indicates that if a mother smokes, her infant may have twice the risk of sudden infant death syndrome (SIDS).

Getting out of harm's way

Steps to limit your exposure to secondhand smoke are straightforward: Stay away from it and keep your children away from it whenever possible.

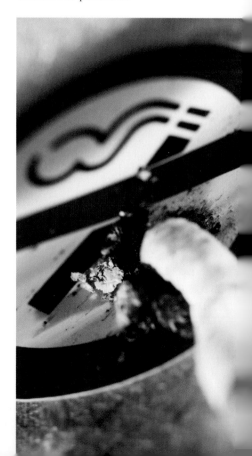

Here are a few specific pointers based on suggestions from the Environmental Protection Agency and the American Lung Association:

- Don't allow smoking inside your home or vehicle. If a family member or guest wants to smoke, ask them to step outside or stop at a rest stop for a smoke break outside the car.

- Choose a smoke-free child care facility. If you take your children to a child care provider, choose one with a no-smoking policy.

- Limit exposure at work. If people are allowed to smoke in your workplace, ask your employer or union to limit or prohibit indoor smoking. Encourage smoking-cessation programs to help your co-workers end their dependence.

- Patronize businesses with no-smoking policies. Support with your business those restaurants and other establishments that have implemented no-smoking policies. When you do have to share a room with people who are smoking, sit as far away from them as possible.

Remember that even if you don't smoke, by being around others who do, you can be putting your health on the same risky path. Don't falsely assume that because you're not the one smoking, your health — or your child's — is in the clear.

Avoiding weight gain

A common fear of many people considering quitting smoking — especially women — is that they'll gain weight. When you stop smoking, your sense of taste and smell return and this may tempt you to eat more. Some people also eat because they're anxious or they don't know what to do with their hands. But quitting doesn't have to mean automatic weight gain. Here are some tips to help you out:

- Eat slowly so your brain can let you know when you're full, and you avoid second helpings. Leave the table as soon as you've finished eating.

- Watch what you eat. At a time when you're battling the urge to eat more, try to keep your meals healthy. More food isn't necessarily a bad thing if it's food that's low in calories, such as vegetables and fruit. Fill up on vegetables and fruit first before eating the rest of your meal.

- If you eat just because you're used to having something in your mouth, chew sugarless gum or snack on foods such as carrots, pickles or celery. Keep your hands busy with things that don't involve food. Play with a "squishy" ball. Or use a straw as a pretend cigarette — something you can hold on to.

- When you have an urge to eat, but you're not truly hungry, get out of the kitchen. Go for a walk, call a friend, take a warm bath, run some errands or clean up the garage.

These suggestions are by no means complete. Test them to find out what works for you and what doesn't.

Step 6
Test Yourself

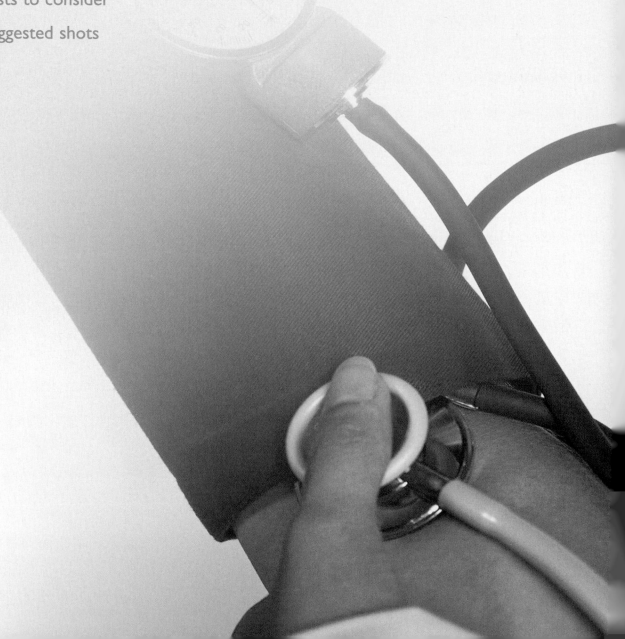

When it comes to preventing illness, there are a couple of strategies you can follow. The primary strategy is to do things that keep a condition from happening in the first place. Take, for example, tobacco use. Research has shown that smoking is a true cause of lung cancer, and so you can prevent lung cancer by not smoking.

The secondary strategy is, once a disease has started, to detect it as early as possible. Screening tests work well for many diseases that exist for a time in an asymptomatic stage — that is, the disease is present in the body but not showing any symptoms. A perfect example is cervical cancer. The infection with the HPV virus can happen early in a woman's life, maybe in her teens or early 20s. The cancer may not develop until 10 years or more after that. So, you have a long period of time to detect the condition — changes on a Pap test generally show up three to five years after the initial infection.

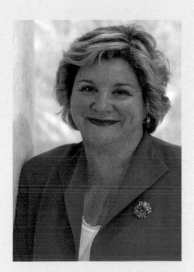

Julie Abbott, M.D.
Preventive Medicine

Whenever a disease can be detected before it becomes symptomatic, for example, vaginal bleeding with cervical cancer, you have the opportunity to prevent it. That's why people should be interested in getting screening tests. It's perhaps the best chance to beat a disease that might otherwise get you.

Expert groups such as the U.S. Preventive Services Task Force have come up with a fairly short list of recommended screening tests. This selection is well founded on evidence and includes the Pap test, mammogram and colorectal screening for cancer. These tests should be considered necessary.

Other tests are commonly done as part of a checkup, but there's little evidence that they're necessary. These include routine urinalysis and annual electrocardiogram. For example, an electrocardiogram may be helpful if you go to the emergency room with chest pains. But it doesn't detect disease, so to have an annual check isn't that useful.

Q: Are regular screening tests all you need for disease prevention?

A: Screening tests are an important part of prevention, but being tested by a doctor is less important than what you yourself can do for prevention. The ball on the court of prevention is your lifestyle. All the decisions you make each day — what you eat, how active you are and what safety precautions you take — that's where the prevention game is really being played. Having screening tests is about a quarter of the action. Three-quarters of the action involves decisions on how you live your life.

Q: What's the most exciting development on the horizon regarding disease prevention?

A: That would have to be the use of genetics for screening and testing. I can't talk about it in great detail because we're still learning so much. But as we come to understand the human genome, we'll be able to truly identify who's going to get a disease and hopefully provide an effective treatment — by altering specific genes — that could change the actual cause and avert your chance of getting sick.

Are you on course?

Health care is a lot like anything else you may be involved in — the more you put in to it, the more you get out of it.

You and your doctor are a team. And it's up to you to work with your doctor to make sure that you receive recommended screenings and immunizations intended to prevent disease, or to catch it early, when the odds for successful treatment are greatest.

Over the next few pages, you'll find information on screening exams, or tests, recommended for people who don't have symptoms or risk factors for a particular medical condition. You'll also find information on additional tests you may want to consider.

Remember, these are general guidelines. If you have risk factors or symptoms, you may need earlier or more frequent testing.

Recommended tests

Following are tests that you should undergo on a regular basis.

Blood cholesterol test

A blood cholesterol test is actually several blood tests (serum lipids). It measures total cholesterol in your blood, as well as the levels of low-density lipoprotein (LDL or "bad") cholesterol, high-density lipoprotein (HDL or "good") cholesterol and other blood fats called triglycerides.

What's the test for?

To measure the levels of cholesterol and triglycerides (lipids) in your blood. Undesirable lipid levels raise your risk of heart attack and stroke. Problems occur when your LDL cholesterol deposits too many fatty deposits on your artery walls or when your HDL cholesterol carries away too few.

When and how often should you have it?

Have a cholesterol evaluation at least every five years if the levels are within normal ranges. If the readings are abnormal, you may have to have your cholesterol checked more often. Cholesterol testing is especially important if you have a family history of high cholesterol or heart disease, are overweight, are physically inactive, have diabetes or eat a high-fat diet. These factors put you at increased risk of developing high cholesterol and heart disease.

Cholesterol by the numbers

Total cholesterol level	Total cholesterol category
Less than 200*	Desirable
200 to 239	Borderline high
240 and above	High

LDL** cholesterol level	LDL cholesterol category
Less than 100	Optimal
100 to 129	Near optimal
130 to 159	Borderline high
160 to 189	High
190 and above	Very high

HDL*** cholesterol level	HDL cholesterol
Less than 40	A major risk factor for heart disease
40 to 59	The higher, the better
60 and above	Protective against heart disease

Triglycerides also can raise your risk of heart disease. Levels that are borderline high (150 to 199 mg/dL) or high (200 mg/dL or more) may require treatment.

Source: National Cholesterol Education Program, 2001

*Numbers are expressed in levels of milligrams of cholesterol per deciliter of blood (mg/dL).

**LDL means low-density lipoprotein.

***HDL means high-density lipoprotein.

Recommended age-specific tests for women

Test	Ages 20-39	Ages 40-50	Older than 50
Blood cholesterol test	Baseline at age 20, then every 5 years	Every 5 years	At least every 5 years
Blood pressure measurement	Every 2 years	Every 2 years	At least every 2 years
Bone density measurement	Ask your doctor	Baseline at menopause	Ask your doctor
Clinical breast exam and mammogram	Ask your doctor; breast exam every 3 years	Ask your doctor; baseline mammogram at age 40	Annually
Colon cancer screening	Ask your doctor	Ask your doctor	Every 5-10 years (depends on test)
Dental checkup	Annually	Annually	Annually
Eye exam	Every 3-5 years, yearly if you wear contacts or glasses	Every 3-5 years, yearly if you wear contacts or glasses	Every 2-4 years, yearly if you wear contacts or glasses
Pap test	Every 1-3 years	Every 1-3 years	Every 1-3 years

Other tests women should consider

Test	Ages 20-39	Ages 40-50	Older than 50
Fasting blood sugar test	Ask your doctor	Baseline by age 45	Every 3 years
Full-body skin exam	Every 3 years	Every 2 years	Annually
Hearing test	Every 10 years	Every 10 years	Every 3 years
Hepatitis screening	Ask your doctor	Ask your doctor	Ask your doctor
Human papillomavirus (HPV)	Ask your doctor	Ask your doctor	Ask your doctor
Thyroid-stimulating hormone test	Ask your doctor	Ask your doctor	Ask your doctor
Transferrin saturation test	Ask your doctor	Ask your doctor	Ask your doctor

Recommended age-specific tests for men

Test	Ages 20-39	Ages 40-50	Older than 50
Blood cholesterol test	Baseline at age 20, then every 5 years	Every 5 years	At least every 5 years
Blood pressure measurement	Every 2 years	Every 2 years	At least every 2 years
Colon cancer screening	Ask your doctor	Ask your doctor	Every 5-10 years (depends on test)
Dental checkup	Annually	Annually	Annually
Eye exam	Every 3-5 years, yearly if you wear contacts or glasses	Every 3-5 years, yearly if you wear contacts or glasses	Every 2-4 years, yearly if you wear contacts or glasses
Prostate-specific antigen (PSA) test and digital rectal exam	Ask your doctor	Ask your doctor	Annually

Other tests men should consider

Test	Ages 20-39	Ages 40-50	Older than 50
Fasting blood sugar test	Ask your doctor	Baseline by age 45	Every 3 years
Full-body skin exam	Every 3 years	Every 2 years	Annually
Hearing test	Every 10 years	Every 10 years	Every 3 years
Hepatitis screening	Ask your doctor	Ask your doctor	Ask your doctor
Thyroid-stimulating hormone test	Ask your doctor	Ask your doctor	Ask your doctor
Transferrin saturation test	Ask your doctor	Ask your doctor	Ask your doctor

What do the numbers mean?

The National Cholesterol Education Program has established guidelines to help determine which numbers are acceptable and which carry increased risk. However, desirable ranges vary depending on your individual health conditions, habits and family history. Talk with your doctor about what cholesterol levels are best for you.

Blood pressure measurement

This test measures the peak pressure your heart generates when pumping blood out through your arteries (systolic blood pressure) and the amount of pressure in your arteries when your heart is at rest between beats (diastolic blood pressure).

What's the test for?

For early detection of high blood pressure. The longer the condition goes undetected and untreated, the higher your risk of heart attack, stroke, heart failure and kidney damage.

When and how often should you have it?

Have your blood pressure checked at least every two years. However, you'll probably have your blood pressure checked every time you see the doctor — whatever the reason. If your blood pressure is borderline or elevated, your doctor may recommend more frequent testing. Blood pressure testing is especially important if you're age 35 or older, black, overweight, inactive or have a family history of high blood pressure. These factors put you at increased risk of developing high blood pressure.

What do the numbers mean?

An ideal or normal blood pressure for an adult of any age is 119 millimeters of mercury (mm Hg) over 79 mm Hg, or lower. This is commonly written as 119/79.

Bone density measurement

This test involves a specialized X-ray scan of your lower back and hip region, wrist or heel.

What's the test for?

To detect osteoporosis — a disease that involves loss of bone mass, making your bones more fragile and likely to break. Osteoporosis especially increases the risk of fractures of your hip, spine and wrist. Several different types of scans are available, including dual energy X-ray absorptiometry (DEXA) and computerized tomography (CT).

When and how often should you have it?

Women should have a baseline exam following menopause. If you have a family history of osteoporosis or other risk factors, earlier testing is a good idea. Risk factors for osteoporosis include early menopause, frequent or extended use of steroid medications, smoking, low body weight, and a history of fractures. Ask your doctor to recommend a testing schedule that's right for you.

What do the numbers mean?

The T-score is a number that describes how much your bone density varies from what's considered normal. "Normal" is based on the typical bone mass in people in their 30s, when bone mass is at its peak.

- T-scores ranging from –1 to +1 or higher mean that your bone density is considered normal and you're at low risk of bone fractures due to osteoporosis.
- T-scores ranging from –2.5 to –1 indicate you have relatively low bone mass .
- T-scores of –2.5 and lower indicate you have osteoporosis and are at greater risk of bone fractures.

Blood pressure by the numbers

Top number (systolic)		Bottom number (diastolic)	Category
119* or lower	and	79 or lower	Normal blood pressure
120 to 139	or	80 to 89	Prehypertension
140 to 159	or	90 to 99	Stage 1 hypertension
160 or more	or	100 or more	Stage 2 hypertension

Source: Seventh Report of the Joint National Committee on Prevention. Detection, Evaluation, and Treatment of High Blood Pressure, 2003

*Numbers are expressed in levels of millimeters of mercury (mm Hg).

Clinical breast exam and mammogram

These two tests are generally done in conjunction with one another.

Clinical breast exam

This is a physical examination of a woman's breast and armpits that's typically part of a routine physical.

What's the test for?

To detect cancer and precancerous changes in the breasts. Your doctor carefully examines your breasts, looking for lumps, color changes, skin irregularities and changes in your nipples. He or she then feels for swollen lymph nodes in the armpits.

When and how often should you have it?

Before age 40, women should have a clinical breast exam at least every three years. For women age 40 and older, the exam should be done every year. Having regular breast exams is particularly important if you have a family history of breast cancer or other factors, including advancing age, which put you at increased risk.

Mammogram

In this screening test, X-rays of your breast tissue are taken while your breasts are compressed between plastic plates.

What's the test for?

To help detect cancer and precancerous changes in female breasts.

Some breast lumps and calcifications, which can be the first indication of early-stage cancer, are too small to be detected on a physical examination.

When and how often should you have it?

Have a baseline mammogram at age 40. Between ages 40 and 49, recommendations vary but you should consider a mammogram every one to two years. Talk with your doctor about what's best for you. Once you turn 50, have a mammogram every year.

If you have a family history of breast cancer, your doctor may recommend that you have mammograms at an earlier age. Regular mammograms also are particularly important if you've had prior abnormal breast biopsies.

If your breasts are sensitive, taking a pain reliever before the test may help ease your discomfort. Avoid using underarm deodorant on the day of your mammogram. It can affect the accuracy of the results.

Colon cancer screening

For this screening exam, a variety of tests may be used. You may have just one or a combination.

- Your stool may be checked for blood (occult blood test).
- You may have an X-ray taken of your colon after an enema with a white, chalky substance that outlines the colon (barium X-ray).
- The inside of your rectum and colon may be examined with a lighted scope (sigmoidoscopy or colonoscopy).

A new technology called virtual colonoscopy is also available in some areas. With virtual colonoscopy, first you undergo a computerized tomography (CT) scan of your colon. Then, using computer imaging, your doctor rotates this X-ray in order to view every part of your colon without actually going inside.

What's the test for?

To detect cancer and growths (polyps) on the inside wall of the colon that could become cancerous (precancerous growths). Many people are afraid to have this test because of fear of embarrassment or discomfort. But this screening could save your life. Removing precancerous polyps can prevent cancer from developing. Early detection of cancer can also be lifesaving.

When and how often should you have it?

If you're at average risk of developing colon cancer, have a screening test every five to 10 years, beginning at age 50. The frequency will depend on the test you have done and your risk of developing the disease. If you're at increased risk of colon cancer, your doctor may recommend beginning screenings earlier.

Dental checkup

Your dentist examines your teeth and checks your tongue, lips, mouth and soft tissues.

What's the test for?

A dental exam is done to detect tooth decay, tooth grinding and diseases such as periodontal disease. Your dentist also looks for lesions and other oral abnormalities that could indicate cancer.

When and how often should you have it?

Have a dental checkup at least once a year or as your dentist recommends.

Regular dental checkups are especially important if your water doesn't contain fluoride or if you use tobacco, regularly drink alcoholic beverages or eat a high-sugar diet.

Eye exam

During the exam, you read eye charts and have your pupils dilated with eyedrops. Your doctor also views the inside of your eye with an instrument called an ophthalmoscope and checks the pressure inside your eyeball with a painless procedure called tonometry.

What's the test for?

An eye exam allows your ophthalmologist or optometrist to check your vision and determine whether you may be at risk of developing vision problems associated with aging, such as glaucoma, cataracts and age-related macular degeneration.

When and how often should you have it?

If you wear glasses or contact lenses, have your eyes checked once a year. If you don't wear corrective lenses, have no eye problems and have no risk factors for eye disease, have your eyes checked every two to four years until age 65. Beginning at age 65, have an eye exam every year or two.

Pap test

In this test, a doctor inserts a speculum into a woman's vagina to observe the cervix. Using a soft brush, he or she gently scrapes a few cells from the cervix, places the cells on a glass slide or in a fluid-filled bottle and sends them to a laboratory for analysis.

What's the test for?

The Pap test detects cancer and precancerous changes in the cervix.

When and how often should you have it?

Women should have a Pap test every one to three years. If you've had normal Pap test results for three years in a row, you and your doctor may opt for a longer interval between tests. For women who've had a total hysterectomy for a noncancerous condition, routine Pap tests aren't necessary.

Getting regular Pap tests is especially important if you smoke or have had a sexually transmitted disease, multiple sex partners or a history of cervical, vaginal or vulvar cancer.

Prostate-specific antigen test and digital rectal exam

During a digital rectal exam, a doctor inserts a lubricated, gloved finger into the male rectum and feels the prostate gland for enlargement, tenderness, lumps or hard spots. The prostate-specific antigen (PSA)

test is a blood test that measures the amount of a specific protein secreted by the male prostate gland.

What are the tests for?

The digital rectal exam can detect prostate enlargement or prostate cancer. Don't be alarmed if your doctor tells you that your prostate gland is enlarged. More than half of men over age 50 have an enlarged prostate caused by a noncancerous condition called benign prostatic hyperplasia (BPH).

With the PSA test, increased levels of PSA may indicate prostate cancer. However, levels can be elevated by BPH or other noncancerous conditions.

When and how often should you have them?

Before age 50, recommendations vary as to when and how often men should have a digital rectal exam and PSA test. Talk with your doctor about what's right for you. Starting at age 50, Mayo Clinic prostate cancer specialists recommend an annual digital rectal exam and PSA test. If you're black or have a family history of prostate cancer, consider beginning screening at an earlier age. These factors put you at increased risk of prostate cancer.

What do the numbers means?

The accompanying age-adjusted scale shows the normal upper PSA limits, based on the PSA test used at Mayo Clinic. Upper limits increase almost every year as you age. If your PSA level is above the normal upper limit for your age, talk with your doctor about what your next step should be.

PSA by the numbers

Age	Upper limit (nanograms/milliliter)
40 or under	2.0
41	2.1
42	2.2
43	2.3
44	2.3
45	2.4
46	2.5
47	2.6
48	2.6
49	2.7
50	2.8
51	2.9
52	3.0
53	3.1
54	3.2
55	3.3
56	3.4
57	3.5
58	3.6
59	3.7
60	3.8
61	4.0
62	4.1
63	4.2
64	4.4
65	4.5
66	4.6
67	4.8
68	4.9
69	5.1
70	5.3
71	5.4
72	5.6
73	5.8
74	6.0
75	6.2
76	6.4
77	6.6
78	6.8
79	7.0
80 or over	7.2

Source: Mayo Clinic

Tests to consider

The tests that follow are recommended for some individuals depending upon their health and their personal risk factors. Talk with your doctor to see if any of these exams may be appropriate for you.

Fasting blood sugar test

This blood test checks for diabetes by measuring the level of sugar (glucose) in your blood after an eight-hour fast.

What's the test for?

High glucose levels can be an indication of diabetes.

When and how often should you have it?

Have a baseline blood glucose test by age 45. If your results are normal, have your blood sugar rechecked every three years. If you have a family history of diabetes or other risk factors for the disease, your doctor may recommend testing at a younger age and more frequently.

What do the numbers mean?

An ideal or normal blood glucose level for an adult of any age is 70 to 100 milligrams of glucose per deciliter of blood (mg/dL).

Full-body skin exam

In this exam, your doctor examines your skin from head to toe, looking for moles that are irregularly shaped, have varied colors, are greater than the size of a pencil eraser, or have grown or changed since the previous visit.

What's the test for?

To check for skin changes associated with skin cancer.

When and how often should you have it?

Have a full-body skin exam every three years in your 20s and 30s. Once you turn 40, have the exam every two years. Once you turn 50, have it every year.

Screening for skin cancer is especially important if you have many moles, fair skin, sun-damaged skin, a family history of skin cancer or had two or more blistering sunburns in childhood. These factors put you at increased risk of skin cancer.

Blood sugar by the numbers

Glucose level	Category
70 to 100 mg/dL*	Normal
101 to 125 mg/dL	Prediabetes**
126 mg/dL or higher on two separate tests	Diabetes

Source: Mayo Clinic

*Numbers are expressed in millimeters of glucose per deciliter of blood (mg/dL).

**Prediabetes means you're at high risk of developing diabetes.

Hearing test

In this test, a doctor checks how well you recognize sounds at various volumes and frequencies.

What's the test for?

To check for hearing loss.

When and how often should you have it?

Check your hearing every 10 years until age 50. At age 50, have it checked every three years.

Hepatitis screening

This is a simple blood test.

What's the test for?

It's used to screen for chronic hepatitis B, C or both, which put you at greater risk of developing liver disease and liver cancer.

When and how often should you have it?

Have a baseline test if you have one or more risk factors. They include having had multiple sex partners, having received a blood transfusion before 1993 and living or traveling in an area where hepatitis B is common.

Human papillomavirus screening

This test is an additional screening option for cervical cancer that may accompany a Pap test.

What's the test for?

This test checks for the presence of a high-risk strain of the human papillomavirus (HPV) in women.

Almost all cervical cancers are linked to infection with a high-risk strain of this virus.

When and how often should you have it?

The HPV test involves the same method used to collect cervical cells during a Pap test. If your Pap test indicates the presence of abnormal cells and you didn't have an accompanying HPV test, you should request one. Although there's no known cure for HPV infection, the cervical changes that result from it can be treated.

Thyroid-stimulating hormone test

This is a simple blood test.

What's the test for?

This test measures the level of thyroid-stimulating hormone (TSH) in your blood, helping to determine if your thyroid may be producing too little (possible hypothyroidism) or too much (possible hyperthyroidism) of a hormone called thyroxine.

When and how often should you have it?

Experts disagree on who may benefit from screening and when it should begin. Talk with your doctor.

Transferrin saturation test

This blood test measures the amount of iron bound to an iron-carrying protein (transferrin) in your bloodstream.

What's the test for?

It can detect iron overload disease, (hemochromatosis), a condition in which your body stores too much iron. Excessive iron can cause organ damage. Hemochromatosis is an underrecognized but treatable hereditary disease.

When and how often should you have it?

Doctors don't regularly test for hemochromatosis, but talk with your doctor about testing if you have a family history of the disease or if you have a condition that can be caused by hemochromatosis. These include heart disease, elevated liver enzymes and diabetes.

Suggested shots

One of the best ways to prevent disease is to make sure you've received all of the recommended immunizations.

Most vaccinations are given in childhood, but some are recommended for adults. Or, perhaps you didn't receive a vaccination in childhood, which could still be of benefit.

The table to the right provides a brief overview of adult immunization recommendations. These are general guidelines. When in doubt, follow your doctor's advice. He or she may recommend that you receive additional vaccinations based on your health status or travel plans.

Recommended immunizations for adults

Disease	What it is	You're at increased risk if:	Doses for adults
Chickenpox (varicella)	A viral disease that spreads easily from person to person, chickenpox is much more serious in adults than in children.	You're a health care worker without immunity or an adult who has never been exposed to the disease or never been vaccinated.	Two-dose series given 4 to 8 weeks apart. Avoid if you have weakened immunity or lymph node or bone marrow cancer, or you've had a serious allergic reaction to gelatin or the antibiotic neomycin.
Hepatitis A	A viral infection of the liver transmitted primarily through contaminated food or water or close personal contact.	You're traveling to a country without clean water or proper sewage, you have chronic liver disease or blood-clotting disorder, use illicit drugs, or are male and homosexual.	Two-dose series with at least 6 months between doses. Avoid if you're hypersensitive to alum or 2-phenoxyethanol, a preservative.
Hepatitis B	A viral infection of the liver that's often transmitted through contaminated blood, sexual contact and prenatal exposure.	You're at occupational risk of exposure to blood and body fluids, are on dialysis or have received blood products, or are sexually active with multiple partners.	Three-dose series given during a 6-month period can prevent this disease. Avoid if allergic to baker's yeast or thimerosal.
Influenza (flu)	A respiratory disease that spreads from person to person by breathing infected droplets from the air.	You're age 50 or older, have a chronic disease, work in health care or have close contact with high-risk people.	One dose every year if you're age 50 or older or in a high-risk group. Avoid if allergic to eggs.
Measles, mumps, rubella	Viral diseases that spread from person to person by breathing infected droplets from the air	You were born after 1956 and don't have proof of previous immunization or immunity.	One or two doses. Avoid if you received blood products in the past 11 months, have weakened immunity or are allergic to the antibiotic neomycin.
Meningo-coccal disease	A disease caused by bacteria or viruses that can cause meningitis, an inflammation of the membranes surrounding the brain and spinal cord.	You have a compromised immune system or you travel to certain foreign countries.	A single dose can prevent a bacterial form of the illness.
Pneumonia	An inflammation of the lungs, which can have various causes, such as bacteria or viruses.	You're age 65 or older, you have a medical condition that increases your risk, such as chronic lung, liver or kidney disease, or you don't have a spleen or it's damaged.	One lifetime dose, but you may need a second dose if you're at higher risk or vaccination was before age 65. Need at least 5 years between doses.
Tetanus and diphtheria	Tetanus is a bacterial infection that develops in deep wounds. Diphtheria is a bacterial infection spread by breathing infected droplets from the air.	You suffer a deep or dirty cut or wound.	Initial three-dose series with booster every 10 years. If your most recent booster was more than 5 years ago, get a booster within 48 hours after a wound.

Step 7
Stay Connected

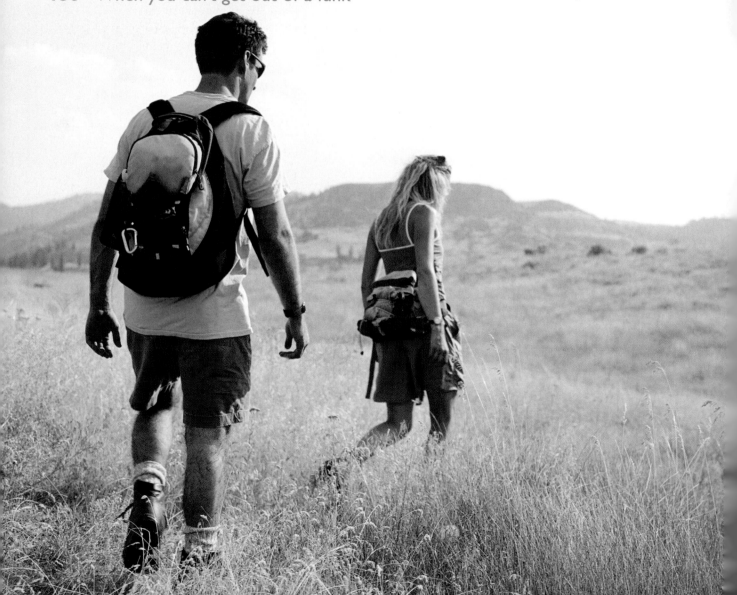

A visit with Dr. Yonas Geda

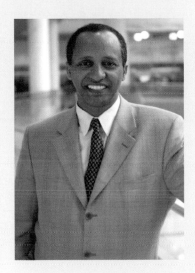

Yonas Geda, M.D.
Psychiatry/Neuropsychiatry

There are obvious reasons why close personal relationships are so important to good health. For starters, the social network that a person belongs to strongly influences lifestyle practices. Hopefully, these influences are positive ones, such as regular physical exercise and not smoking. As well, a person often benefits from the unconditional acceptance that results from stable social relationships — bolstering self-confidence, motivation and a positive outlook.

Having said this, you should be cautious of studies that make a direct association between social networks and longevity. These risk estimates are for groups of people and may not apply to every individual. You don't have to be exceedingly social in order to live long — I'm sure we can all think of a quiet, reserved person who has led a long, contented life. Another caution is that not all relationships are healthy and, in fact, some can be quite harmful to your health. A key issue for you will be judging whether you're in a relationship that contributes to your physical and spiritual well-being.

Why do so many people discount the effects of emotions and personal relationships on their health? At this point, we can only speculate because much of what we know about the brain has been revealed only in the last 10 to 20 years. Before this, people tended to treat the physical brain and the intellectual mind almost as separate and somewhat unrelated entities, obscuring the connections between physical health and the emotions.

Then, there's the stigma associated with emotional behavior. Think of your emotions on a spectrum, with one end being positive and the other end being extreme and pathological. Consider something like anxiety, for example. A little anxiety can be positive — preparing you for an exam or motivating you to meet a deadline — but too much anxiety will incapacitate you. People tend to associate emotional behavior with the negative end of the spectrum, while ignoring positive aspects at the other end.

Q: Why are people encouraged to 'stay connected' when relationships can be a major source of stress and conflict?

A: You must strive for relationships that are stable, reciprocal and nuturing, but that's easier said than done. We can't always control with whom we associate. For example, you can't determine whether you get a good boss or a cranky boss. What you can do is work on how you approach the relationship. You can try to approach it patiently, calmly and in a thoughtful manner. Or you can approach it impulsively, frantically or in anger. Getting something positive from a difficult relationship is extremely hard work.

Q: Do pessimism and depression tend to go hand in hand?

A: Pessimism simply means being adept at viewing the negative aspects of a situation by discounting the positive or neutral aspects. It's a kind of slate on which someone's general outlook is written. A pessimistic outlook can make someone vulnerable to depression, but the two are not identical. Depression has biological and psychosocial symptoms that can be fatal (by suicide) in a severe state.

Relationships:
A prescription for better health

You can't imagine what life would be like without your spouse or your best friend. He or she makes you laugh, and always provides a listening ear when you need one. Did you know these individuals also may be keeping you healthy?

Relationships play a vital role in overall health and happiness. Throughout life, a healthy marriage, good friendships and strong family ties contribute to mental and emotional well-being.

Studies also show that people who enjoy social support — close ties with family, friends and partners — tend to not only be healthier but live longer.

Vital connections

Increasing evidence suggests that physical factors such as your blood pressure level and your immune system could be affected by psychosocial factors, things such as your attitude and your relationships.

Whereas social isolation is known to contribute to illness and poor health, strong social connections appear to boost your health in a number of ways:

Bolster immunity

It's clear that stress can suppress immunity. To the contrary, love and friendship reduce stress and strengthen immunity. One study found that people with more diverse social networks were less susceptible to the common cold.

Improve mental health

Having other people to talk with during difficult times provides a psychological buffer against stress, anxiety and depression.

Even when you don't have a crisis in your life, social networks increase your sense of belonging, purpose and self-worth, promoting positive mental health. Healthy relationships also help reduce anxiety.

Improve recovery

Researchers who reviewed more than 50 studies examining the link between social support and cardiovascular disease concluded that individuals who don't have strong social support have worse recovery after a heart attack.

In fact, lack of social support appears to be as harmful as other cardiovascular risk factors, including high cholesterol, smoking and high blood pressure.

People with a strong support system likely recover faster because they're more motivated to do so, they're more likely to adhere to treatment regimens and their risk of depression is reduced.

Protect against mental decline

Individuals who frequently interact with larger networks — be it extended family, or civic and church groups — generally maintain better mental sharpness (acuity) over time.

Extend life

More than a dozen studies link social support with a lower risk of early death. In one study, researchers monitored the health of nearly 7,000 Californians for more than 17 years. They found that those who were more isolated — who lacked social connections — were two to three times as likely to die younger as were their more socially connected counterparts.

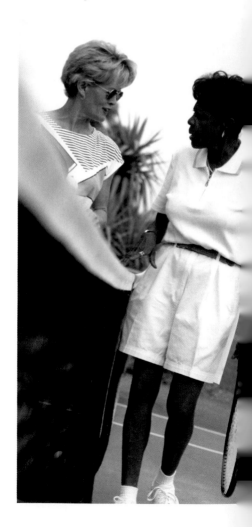

Widening your circle

If you feel that your social network is too small, remember that you can always branch out. Here are some ways to make new connections and to maintain existing ones:

Make relationships a priority

One of the best support sources is a healthy, fulfilling long-term relationship. Don't take your spouse or partner for granted. Take time to be there for each other. In addition, make time to regularly do something with your friends so that they know you're invested in the friendship.

Know the importance of give and take

Sometimes you're the one giving support and other times you're on the receiving end. Recognize who is able to provide you with the most support. Letting family and friends know you love and appreciate them will help ensure that their support remains strong when times are rough.

Respect boundaries

Although you want to be there for friends and family, you don't want to overwhelm them either. Respect their ways of communicating. Find out how late or early you can call or how often they like to get together.

It's never too late to make new friends

It's always fun to meet new people and develop new friendships. Doing so doesn't have to be difficult.

- **Get out with your pet.** Seek out a park or make conversation with those who stop to talk.

- **Try new things with your children.** Sign your children up for an activity, or take them on an outing to a new park or museum. Taking part in activities with your children is a great way to meet new friends.

- **Work out.** Join a lunchtime walking group at work. Sign up for a class through a local gym or community fitness facility.

- **Volunteer.** Hospitals, churches, museums, community centers and other organizations often need volunteers. You can form strong connections when you work with people who have a mutual goal.

- **Join a cause.** Get together with a group of people working toward a goal you believe in, such as an election campaign or the cleanup of a natural resources area.

- **Find a hobby group.** If you have a particular hobby, check to see if there's a group of people in your community with similar interests.

- **Take a class.** A college or community education course can put you in touch with people who have similar interests.

Listen up

Make a point to listen to others and be aware of what's going on in their lives.

Be aware of how others perceive you

Ask a friend for an honest evaluation of how you come across to others. Take note of any areas for improvement and work on them.

Don't compete with others

Competition can turn potential friends into potential rivals. Try to be noncompetitive.

Adopt a healthy, realistic self-image

Both vanity and rampant self criticism can be unattractive. Nurture those qualities that you enjoy in others.

Adopt a positive outlook

Try to take a positive view — instead of always a negative one — of situations at hand. Persistent pessimism or nonstop complaining is tiresome and can be draining on support systems.

When appropriate, look for the humor in things.

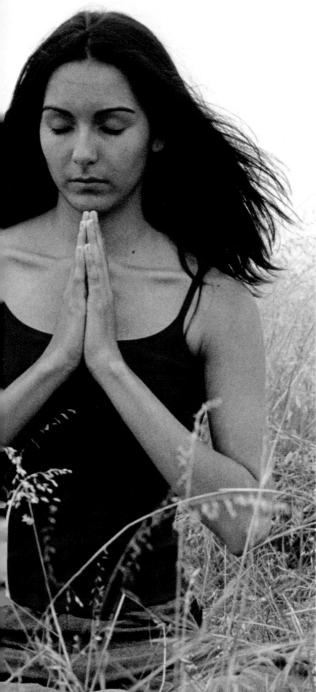

Believing in a higher power

Similar to the benefits that come from strong ties with family and friends, spiritual bonds also promote good health. Spiritual well-being can have a positive influence on your health and happiness.

Defining spirituality

People often use the word *spirituality* interchangeably with *religion*. Although there's considerable overlap between the two concepts, the terms aren't necessarily synonymous. While religion typically refers to a formal system of beliefs, attitudes or practices held by a group of believers, spirituality is more individualistic and self-determined. There may be as many definitions of spirituality as there are people in the world. One definition commonly used is "a personal search for meaning and purpose in life."

Both spirituality and religion prompt you to turn inward and reflect on your own life and its purpose. Your spiritual beliefs can help you prioritize your life and develop interests that have the potential to be most fulfilling. At the same time, spiritual beliefs and practices help you to connect to something greater than yourself.

Vital connections

More studies are suggesting that when you believe in some form of higher power, you strengthen your ability to cope with whatever life hands you.

At least one study found that people who regularly attend religious services tend to enjoy better health, live longer and recover from illness faster and with fewer complications than those who don't attend religious services. Individuals who attend religious services also tend to cope better with illness and experience less depression.

What's the link?

Researchers aren't quite sure of the mechanisms through which religion and spirituality promote mental and physical health. Some factors thought to play a role include:

Social support
Whether you attend a church, synagogue or mosque, these religious settings usually have a built-in social support structure that's readily available to its members. And as you just read, social support has many positive effects on health.

Coping resources

Your religious beliefs may help you make sense of the world around you and the crises and tragedies that arise. Turning to a higher power for comfort and strength may provide relief from stressors that can have a negative impact on health. Belief in something greater than yourself also may help you to accept and cope with events that are beyond your control.

In addition, the feeling of hope, prominent in many faiths, may boost your immune system.

Social values

Research suggests that people who belong to religious organizations are less likely to smoke or abuse alcohol or drugs, more inclined to view physical activity as a priority, and less likely to carry or use weapons, get into fights and engage in risky sexual behavior than are those who are less religious.

Forgiveness

The practice of forgiveness is prominent in religion. There's evidence that forgiving others promotes mental and physical well-being, possibly by:

- Alleviating the forgiver of the burden of pent-up anger and resentment
- Re-establishing social ties that may have been a major source of support
- Promoting positive emotions, which can reduce anxiety and reduce blood pressure

Prayer

Engaging in ritual activities, such as prayer, promotes relaxation, which is characterized by lowered blood pressure, heart rate and breathing rate. This may have a protective effect, particularly against high blood pressure.

Research on prayer has also revealed some other interesting findings over the years.

- Sitting quietly and thinking about God (meditative prayer) is more likely to promote relaxation than is asking God for something specific (petitionary prayer) or reciting prayers (ritual prayer).
- Praying for others enhances self-esteem because it takes your mind off your own troubles, and it allows you to feel as if you're helping someone in need.
- Feelings of self-worth are highest among individuals who believe that God answers prayer at the best time and in the best way, as opposed to those who believe their prayers are answered immediately and in exactly the manner that they requested.

A healthy spirit, a healthy body

Research suggests religion and spirituality promote good health the following ways:

Physical health

- Longer life
- Less cardiovascular disease and fewer deaths from cardiovascular disease
- Lower blood pressure
- Better immune function
- Healthy behaviors: more exercise, better nutrition, better sleep, less smoking, increased use of seat belts and preventive health services
- Fewer hospitalizations and shorter hospital stays

Mental health

- Less risk of depression and better recovery from depression
- Less anxiety and more rapid recovery from anxiety disorders
- Less substance abuse
- Decreased risk of suicide
- Greater well-being, hope and optimism
- More purpose and meaning in life
- Greater marital satisfaction and stability
- Greater social support

Adapted from Koenig, H.G., "Religion, Spirituality, and Medicine: Research Findings and Implications for Clinical Practice, *Southern Medical Journal*, December 2004; and Mueller, P.S., et al, "Religious Involvement, Spirituality, and Medicine: Implications for Clinical Practice," *Mayo Clinic Proceedings*, December 2001

Is your attitude harming your health?

As you make your way through life and the various transitions it brings, you'll find that an optimistic attitude — along with strong social and spiritual connections — can make your days more enjoyable and less stressful. Your attitude may also affect how long you'll live.

Optimists live longer

Increasing evidence suggests that being an optimist or a pessimist affects your health. A recent Dutch study found that adults with an optimistic disposition — people who generally expected good things to happen rather than bad things — lived longer than those who tended to expect doom and gloom.

At the beginning of the study, more than 900 participants completed surveys that assessed their well-being, including their sense of optimism. Those who scored high on the optimism scale had a 29 percent lower risk of early death than did participants who scored low.

Optimism appeared to be particularly protective against death from cardiovascular disorders. Highly optimistic participants were 77 percent less likely to die of a heart attack, stroke or other cardiovascular event than were highly pessimistic participants. This was true regardless of whether they had a history of cardiovascular disease or high blood pressure.

A study conducted at Mayo Clinic produced similar results. In this study, researchers examined the relationship between explanatory styles — how individuals explained the causes of life's events — of more than 800 participants. And then they tracked the group's death rate during a 30-year period.

The researchers found that individuals who had a more pessimistic explanatory style died younger than those whose style was more optimistic.

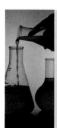

A recent Mayo Clinic study found that pessimists and people with depression have a 30 percent increased risk of developing dementia several decades later. The higher the scores on the pessimism and depression scales, the higher was the risk of dementia.

Mayo researchers caution, though, about jumping to conclusions. More research is needed, and people who consider themselves to be pessimists or who may be depressed shouldn't think they're on a one-way course for dementia.

Optimists tended to believe the causes of bad events were temporary, not their fault and limited to present circumstances. Pessimists, meanwhile, tended to blame things on themselves, feel bad situations would last forever and worry a bad event would undermine everything.

Optimists live better

Thirty years after they filled out the original questionnaire, Mayo researchers asked the same group of participants a series of questions relating to their physical and mental health.

Optimists reported fewer health limitations, fewer problems with work or other daily routines, less pain, more energy, and feeling more peaceful, happier and calmer most of the time.

To the contrary, studies suggest pessimists are prone to depression, have a weakened immune system and use health care services more frequently.

What's the link?

Scientists aren't sure how optimism promotes better health. It's possible optimists cope more effectively with life events and have healthier habits that are more likely to promote recovery. There also may be biological differences involving factors such as the immune system, genetics, hormones and heart rate.

Judging life — and yourself

People generally don't choose to be optimists or pessimists. The attitude you take toward life events is likely a combination of genetics, early environment and life experiences. If your parents tended to be more pessimistic than optimistic, you may be, too.

But that doesn't mean you're stuck with your attitude. Pessimism may be changeable to some degree. Granted, you may not be able to transform yourself into someone with an eternally upbeat view of life, but by being mindful of the ways in which your viewpoint brings you down or influences how you think, you may be able to view some events in a different manner.

Instead of seeing life from just one vantage point, try to acquire the skill of viewing the positive, negative and neutral aspects of life events. Like all new skills, this requires practice and hard work. Here are some suggestions:

- **Be aware of negative thoughts.** Pay attention to the messages you give yourself. When you catch yourself thinking that life is terrible, tell yourself this is only one way of looking at life.

- **Put things in perspective.** Some people are so negative that even when small things go wrong, they feel as if they're cursed. Remember, everyone has ups and downs and nobody's life is perfect.

- **Try reframing.** Reframing can help you find the good in a bad situation. For example, if you've lost your job, acknowledge the feeling of loss. Then, when you're ready, try to look for the positive in the situation. You might ask yourself, "Could I take this as an opportunity to learn a new skill?"

- **Count your blessings.** Gratitude can help you focus on what's right in your life. Look around you and make a mental list of all the things you take for granted but for which you are truly grateful.

- **Forgive and let go.** Learn from your mistakes, forgive yourself and move on. Also forgive others. Hanging on to a hurt or a wrong done to you by someone else only gives that hurt more power over you.

- **Savor the good times.** Good memories can get you through the bad times. Savor those moments when all is well.

- **Pursue simple pleasures.** If you find satisfaction in the small things in life — a relaxing cup of coffee or time spent with friends — you won't need spectacular events to be happy.

- **Be kind.** Being kind to friends and strangers can relieve some of the tension in their lives and make you feel better about your own.

When you can't get out of a funk

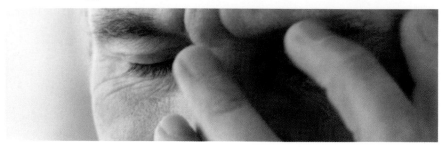

Sometimes, try as you may, you can't achieve that optimistic edge or muster up the energy to reach out to friends and family. Something seems to be zapping your energy, skewing your outlook and taking the fun out of life. Is it possible you may be depressed?

Depression affects more than 18 million Americans of all ages and races. It's a disorder that influences your thoughts, moods, feelings, behaviors and physical health. People used to think depression was "all in your head" and that if you really tried, you could "pull yourself out of it." Not true. Depression isn't a weakness, and you can't treat it on your own. It's a medical disorder with a biological or chemical basis.

Sometimes, a stressful life event triggers depression. Other times it seems to occur spontaneously with no identifiable specific cause. Occasionally, people experience bouts of depression and aren't even aware of it.

Warning signs

Two hallmarks of depression are:

- **Loss of interest in normal daily activities.** You lose interest in or pleasure from activities that you used to enjoy. This condition is called anhedonia.
- **Depressed mood.** You feel sad, helpless or hopeless, and may have crying spells.

In addition to these features, for a doctor or other health professional to make a diagnosis of depression, most of the following signs and symptoms also must be present nearly every day for at least two weeks:

- **Sleep disturbances.** Sleeping too much or having difficulty sleeping can be a sign that you're depressed. Waking up in the middle of the night or early in the morning and not being able to fall back to sleep are typical.
- **Impaired thinking or concentration.** You may have trouble concentrating or making decisions. You may also have more difficulty remembering things.
- **Significant weight loss or gain.** An increased or reduced appetite and unexplained weight gain or loss may indicate depression.
- **Agitation or slowing of body movements.** You may seem restless, agitated, irritable and easily annoyed. Or you may seem to do everything in slow motion and answer questions slowly in a monotonous tone of voice.
- **Fatigue.** You feel weariness and lack of energy nearly every day. You may feel as tired in the morning as you did when you went to bed the night before.

- **Low self-esteem.** You may feel worthless and have excessive guilt.
- **Less interest in sex.** If you were sexually active before developing depression, you may notice a dramatic decrease in your level of interest in having sexual relations.
- **Thoughts of death.** You have a persistent negative view of yourself, your situation and the future. You may have thoughts of death, dying or suicide.

Depression can also cause a variety of physical complaints, such as generalized itching, blurred vision, excessive sweating, gastrointestinal problems, headache and backache.

Children, teens and older adults may react differently. In these groups, symptoms may take different forms or may be masked by other conditions.

If you experience any of the symptoms discussed — especially if you find that you're no longer interested in activities you once enjoyed, or if you often feel sad, helpless or worthless — see your doctor. The sooner depression is identified, often the easier it is to treat. Your doctor can refer you to appropriate experts.

Women and depression: Understanding the gender gap

Nearly twice as many women as men develop depression-related disorders at some point in their lives. What's behind this apparent gender gap?

Biological factors

Among females, hormones may alter mood through various stages of life. It's after puberty that the gender disparity in depression-related disorders truly becomes pronounced.

Premenstrual problems

For most women, symptoms that often occur before menstruation — anxiety, irritability or a blue mood — are minor and short-lived. But a small percentage of women have severe premenstrual symptoms, including depression and hopelessness, known as pre-menstrual dysphoric disorder (PMDD). Cyclical changes in estro-gen and other hormones may severely disrupt those brain chemi-cals that control mood, causing PMDD. However, because hor-monal changes occur in all women, but not all women develop depres-sion, other factors likely play a role.

Pregnancy

Dramatic hormonal changes dur-ing pregnancy, along with life, work and relationship changes, may trig-ger depression. Other factors that can increase the risk of depression during pregnancy include previous depression or PMDD, marital strife, insufficient social support and ambivalence about being pregnant. It can be difficult to

recognize depression during preg-nancy because its symptoms can mimic normal changes associated with pregnancy.

Postpartum depression

About half of women find them-selves sad, irritable and prone to tears soon after giving birth. These feelings, often called the baby blues, are normal and generally subside within a week or two. If they don't or if the symptoms are severe — especially if they're cou-pled with feelings of anxiety, low self-esteem, agitation or thoughts of suicide — you might have post-partum depression. Postpartum depression isn't merely a matter of being unable to cope with a new baby, but is likely associated with major hormonal fluctuations that influence mood.

Perimenopause and menopause

Risk of depression can increase during the transition to meno-pause (perimenopause), when hormone levels fluctuate erratical-ly, as well as after menopause, when estrogen levels are signifi-cantly reduced. For women whose sleep is disrupted for long periods or who have a prior history of depression, this can be a vulnera-ble time.

Social and cultural factors

It's not just biology that may account for the higher rate of depression in women. Other factors play a role, too.

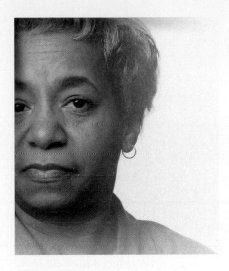

Unequal power and status

Single women with children have one of the highest poverty rates in the United States. Minority women may also face stress from racial discrimination. These issues can contribute to feelings of nega-tivism and lack of self-esteem, which increase risk of depression.

Work overload

Many women work outside the home but still handle the bulk of domestic chores. They often log more hours each week than do men attending to the needs of others. In addition, women often find themselves sandwiched between generations — caring for their young children while also caring for sick and older family members. These kinds of stresses may make you vulnerable to depression.

Sexual and physical abuse

Women who were sexually molested or otherwise abused as children or teenagers are more likely to experience depression at some point in their lives. Adult women who experience abuse — physical, emotional, sexual — are also at greater risk of depression.

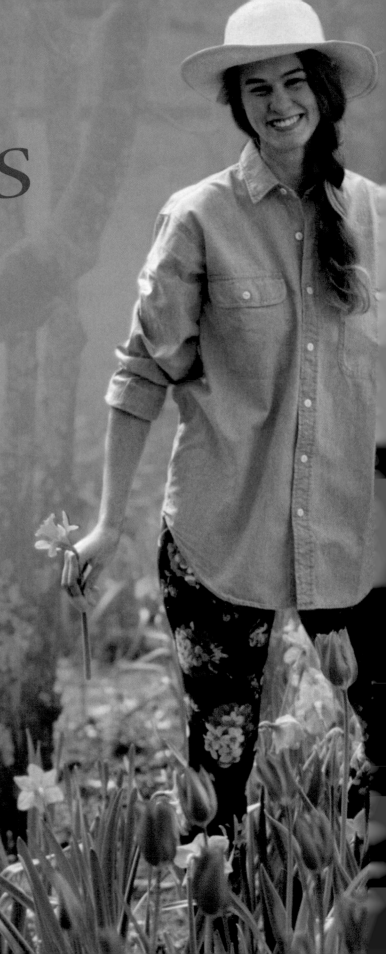

Step 8
Address Stress

A visit with Dr. Kristin Vickers Douglas

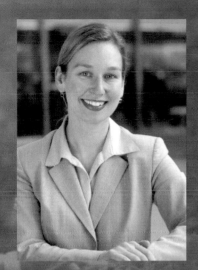

Kristin Vickers Douglas, Ph.D.
Psychiatry & Psychology

As a clinical psychologist at Mayo Clinic, I work with many adults who are experiencing the negative consequences of stress, and are at a point of feeling quite overwhelmed. Often, these same people are very good at taking care of the needs of others — many are health care providers, parents, or in some other helping profession. Although they may have wonderful skills for taking care of others, I see them putting their own self-care at a low priority. I tell them, "You can take care of others better when you take care of yourself."

Managing stress is important to our physical and emotional well-being and should be an active and ongoing process, not just a set of strategies for use in difficult times. Too often we wait until a stressful situation is out of control before taking action.

If I'm stressed, the first thing to go is my sleep. I'll wake up early in the morning and think of all the things that I need to do. I'll also notice muscle tension, typically in my neck and in my back. Paying attention to my body and knowing my early signs of increasing stress help me recognize the need to take action. I then make a conscious effort to use stress management strategies, such as those discussed on the following pages. It's important not to passively wait for stressful situations to resolve. Active use of stress management strategies can help us manage symptoms of stress while meeting other important obligations in our lives.

Q: Is it true that stress can cause you to age faster?

A: When describing the impact of ongoing stress in their lives, my patients often say something like, "It feels like I've aged 10 years in the last several months." Some preliminary research suggests that stress may indeed impact aging at the cellular level. Additionally, we know that, when under stress, people often discontinue use of the health behaviors that could help them better manage their stress. People with high levels of stress report higher rates of smoking, making unhealthy food choices, avoiding exercise, and insufficient sleep. Stress and avoidance of healthy behaviors can result in feelings of fatigue, greater susceptibility to illness, and an overall sense of poor health.

Q: Do you have a preferred method for coping with stress?

A: I find that I have to get back to basics when I'm under stress. Like many, I'm prone to skipping healthy behaviors when I'm feeling stressed, because it seems other things are more important. However, I know that if I skip meals, sleep less, and avoid exercise, I'm less effective in managing my stressors. My favorite stress-relieving strategies include going for walks, pleasant distractions such as a good movie or book, and social support — especially from someone who can make me laugh. I also try to prevent stress by setting limits on demands for my time, especially when I'm feeling overwhelmed. Although I sometimes find it unpleasant to say no to requests, I've learned that I can be most productive and successful when I set healthy limits.

I encourage my patients to cope with their stress by trying a variety of stress management approaches to find the ones that work best for them — emphasizing that stress management should be practiced daily, not just in times of extreme distress.

Feelin' stressed?

Modern-day life is stressful — it's full of pressure and frustration. Heavy workloads, a demanding family life, aging parents — these situations and countless others can cause you to feel pressured, worn-out and unable to keep up.

Stress is a normal part of everyday life, but you don't have to let stress get the best of you.

Understanding stress

Stress doesn't result from specific life events. It's your personal response to certain situations that produces stress. That's why an event that may be stressful to you, such as driving in heavy traffic, isn't to someone else.

Stress can be short term (acute) or long term (chronic).

Acute stress is the stress you experience during an immediate or perceived threat. In such cases, your body responds with an alarm reaction that prepares you for an emergency. It generates a physical response to meet the energy demands of the situation. Once the threat passes, your body relaxes again.

Chronic stress stems from situations that aren't short lived, such as relationship problems or financial worries. Your physical response may not be as extreme but your body is in a stressful state for a longer period of time.

Your body can handle an occasional stressful event, but when you experience stress on a regular basis, its effects can compound over time. The result is a toll on your health.

Common causes

Long workdays, too little sleep and information overload are among the leading sources of stress. However, situations that create stress are as unique as you are.

Your personality, genes and past experiences — your overall ability to cope — influence how you deal with stressful situations. Missing the bus, standing in line at the store or getting a parking ticket may not bother you, but another person may find these situations extremely stressful.

Studies suggest life experiences can increase your sensitivity to stress. People who were exposed to significant stress as children tend to be particularly vulnerable to stress as adults.

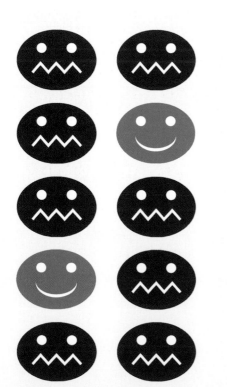

Living with too much stress

In a recent national survey, eight of 10 Americans indicated they had measurable stress in their lives, and more than half of respondents said their stress level was higher than they wanted it to be.

What has Americans stressed out?

- 74 percent said they were worried about their health and the health of their family.

- 70 percent said they were concerned about their family finances.

- 68 percent said they were concerned about their safety and their family's safety.

- 58 percent said they don't get enough sleep.

- 41 percent said they were burned out and overloaded with work.

- 25 percent said they were overextended and involved in too many organizations or activities.

Stress in action

Many of the physical reactions that accompany stress can damage your long-term health. Stress may be a factor in a variety of illnesses, from headaches to heart disease. Stress may aggravate an existing health problem, or it may trigger an illness if you're already at risk of that particular condition.

Suppresses the immune system

The hormone cortisol produced during the stress response can suppress your immune system, increasing your susceptibility to infections. Studies suggest that the risk of bacterial infections such as tuberculosis and group A streptococcal disease increases during stress. Stress may also make you prone to upper respiratory viral infections such as a cold or the flu.

Increases risk of cardiovascular disease

During acute stress your heart beats quickly, making you more susceptible to heart-rhythm irregularities and a type of chest pain called angina. What's more, if you're a "hot reactor," acute stress may add to your risk of a heart attack. Hot reactors exhibit extreme increases in heart rate and blood pressure in response to daily stress. These surges may gradually injure your coronary arteries and heart. Increased blood clotting from persistent stress also can put you at risk of a heart attack or stroke.

Worsens other illnesses

Other relationships between illness and stress aren't as clear-cut. However, stress may worsen your symptoms if you have any of the following conditions:

Asthma

A stressful situation can make your airways overreactive, precipitating an asthma attack.

Gastrointestinal problems

Stress may trigger or worsen symptoms associated with some gastrointestinal conditions, such as irritable bowel syndrome or nonulcer dyspepsia.

Skin disorders

Stress can worsen some skin disorders such as psoriasis, eczema, hives and acne.

Chronic pain

Stress can heighten your body's pain response, making chronic pain associated with conditions such as arthritis or a back injury more difficult to manage.

Mental health disorders

Stress may trigger depression in people who are prone to the disorder. It may also worsen symptoms of other mental health disorders, such as anxiety.

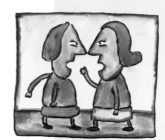

The good side of stress

Not all stress is bad. Stress can result from both negative and positive situations. Negative stress occurs when you feel out of control or under constant or intense pressure. Finances, isolation and health problems are common causes of negative stress. Stress brought on by a positive cause — such as the birth of a child or a new job — provides a feeling of excitement and opportunity. Positive stress helps challenge and motivate us.

Researchers surveying 30 years of studies on stress found that short-lived (acute) stress — stress that has an end in sight — may actually boost your immune system. Stress can also be mentally stimulating. Life without any stress can be boring, whereas a tolerable amount of stress can make a challenging task exciting and increase productivity and chances for success. For example, stress often helps athletes perform better in competition.

Other studies suggest that "good" stress may trigger a cascade of cellular events resulting in the repair or elimination of damaged cellular proteins. This may help prevent cell damage, which, in turn, helps prevent disease and promotes longevity.

Stress isn't always easy to recognize

You may not realize that you're under stress. Your first indications that your body and brain are feeling pressured may be more common symptoms of stress — headache, insomnia, upset stomach, digestive changes. An old nervous habit such as nail biting may reappear. But instead of recognizing these symptoms as stress, you may at first interpret them as an illness.

Stress can also produce psychological changes. The most common is increased irritability with people close to you. You may also feel more cynical, pessimistic or resentful. You may find things you normally enjoyed now seem burdensome. Sometimes, these changes are so gradual that you or those around you don't recognize them.

Signs and symptoms of stress

Physical	Psychological	Behavioral
Headache	Anxiety	Overeating or loss of appetite
Grinding teeth	Irritability	Impatience
Tight, dry throat	Feeling of impending doom	Being argumentative
Clenched jaws	Depression	Procrastination
Chest pain	Slowed thinking	Increased use of alcohol or drugs
Shortness of breath	Racing thoughts	Increased smoking
Pounding heart	Feeling of helplessness	Withdrawal or isolation
High blood pressure	Feeling of hopelessness	Neglecting responsibility
Muscle aches	Feeling of worthlessness	Poor job performance
Indigestion	Feeling of lack of direction	Burnout
Constipation or diarrhea	Feeling of insecurity	Poor personal hygiene
Increased perspiration	Sadness	Change in religious practices
Cold, sweaty hands	Defensiveness	Change in close relationships
Fatigue	Anger	
Insomnia	Hypersensitivity	
Frequent illness	Apathy	

10 ways to stress less

There are many ways to deal with stress. You may talk about your problems with others, listen to some music to help you relax, or sit in a warm bathtub or hot tub at the end of the day. Much of this you do without really thinking about it.

Most of the time you may do pretty well in getting through life's crises as they arise. However, there are probably times when you could do better. The following strategies can help you better manage stress.

#1. Identify your stressors

The first step in learning to manage stress is to identify what's causing it.

Stress may be linked to external factors, such as:

- Work
- Family
- Community
- Environment
- Unpredictable events

Stress can also come from internal factors, such as:

- Unrealistic or high expectations
- Perfectionism
- Worry
- Negative attitudes and feelings
- Irresponsible behavior
- Poor health and health habits

Once you identify the sources of your stress, you might not be able to avoid them, but you'll at least know what's causing your symptoms. That in itself may be a benefit by making you feel more in control.

#2. Develop an action plan

Once you've identified your stressors and have accepted that they exist, it's time to address them.

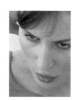

Some stressors are under your control; others aren't. Concentrate on events that you can change. For example, if your busy day is a source of stress, ask yourself if it's because you tend to squeeze too many things into your day or because you aren't organized. Here are some tips that may help:

Simplify your life

Stress often is the result of cramming too much activity into too little time. Rather than trying to find a way to fit everything in, try to find a way to leave some things out. Prioritize, plan and pace yourself.

Plan your day

Planning your day can help you feel more in control of your life. Keep a schedule of your daily activities so that you're not faced with conflicts or last-minute rushes to get to an appointment or activity on time.

Get organized

Organize your home and work space so that you don't have to spend time looking for things you've misplaced.

Exercise

Exercise is one of the best tools there is for managing stress. People who exercise are better able to cope with stress and less likely to become depressed or anxious. While exercise may be physically demanding, it's mentally relaxing and soothing.

#3. Practice tolerance

Try to become more tolerant of yourself and of situations over which you have no control. You need to understand and accept that changes are constant and that certain changes — losses, disappointments and events over which you may have little control — will continue to occur, like it or not.

If you're like most people, you're more understanding of other people's distress than of your own. You may think that you should always feel happy. As long as you believe this, you're bound to be disappointed. Accept that you'll always experience a certain degree of stress, and that this is normal.

#4. Learn to manage anger

Anger management is an important technique for reducing stress. Anger can significantly

Putting time on your side

Often, stress is a result of too much to do and too little time to do it. Or it may stem from procrastination. Setting priorities and practicing some simple time management skills can go a long way toward depressurizing your day.

1. Dump all of your tasks onto a master list. Include everything you have to do, large and small. You may have 50 items. Mark key dates and deadlines for big projects on your calendar.

2. Each day, list five to 10 items that you want to accomplish that day.

3. Divide your daily list into three levels — A, B and C:

- A items are the two or three tasks that you must do. These tasks are both important and urgent and probably will take the most energy. Do them first or when your energy level is the highest.

- B items are important but not urgent. These activities will help you move toward your long-range goals.

- C items are routine stuff, but things that you must do today. Can you delegate any of these?

If you're still having problems getting the things done, analyze how you spend your time for several days. You may be wasting time on unimportant things or things that aren't on your list.

increase and prolong stress if you remain angry for an extended period. Anger can even trigger a heart attack. Learning to manage anger is a lot like learning to manage stress. Here are some suggestions to help you get started:

Identify your anger triggers

Once you know what sets you off, plan ahead for how you'll avoid becoming angry when you're in such a situation.

Identify symptoms of emerging anger

What do you do when you start to get angry? Do you clench your teeth? Do your shoulders begin to tense up? Do you feel your heart begin to beat faster? Does your face flush? Read these signs and symptoms like a caution light — a warning that you're getting angry.

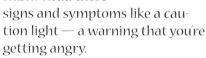

Respond to your symptoms

When you find yourself becoming angry, take a short timeout. Count to 10, take a few deep breaths, look out a window — anything to buy time so that your brain can catch up with your emotions and you can think before you act.

Take time to cool down

Before you confront a person or situation that has made you angry, find a way to release some of your emotional energy. Go for a walk or run, or clean the house. And don't hit the send button on that angry e-mail you just wrote.

Don't bottle up your anger

If your anger stems from what someone said or did, talk directly to that person. Don't verbally attack the person with accusations. Deal only with this episode and approach it from the perspective of how you feel instead of what the person did.

Find release valves

Look for creative ways to release the energy produced by your anger. These might include listening to music, painting, dancing or writing in your journal.

Seek advice

If you find yourself becoming angry often, confide in people who care about you, such as family members or friends. Ask them to help you brainstorm possible coping solutions or find a medical professional who can help you learn to manage your anger.

#5. Practice positive thinking

Positive self-talk is another effective way to cope with stress. Self-talk is the endless stream of thoughts that run through your head every day. These automatic thoughts can be positive or negative. Some are based on logic and reason. Others may be misconceptions. More often than not, our thoughts cause us to worry unnecessarily.

The goal of positive self-talk is to weed out the misconceptions and challenge them with rational and positive thoughts. Studies indicate that a positive, hopeful attitude can help manage stress, but a negative attitude can aggravate it.

How can you learn positive self-talk? The process is simple, but it takes time and practice. Throughout the day, stop and evaluate what you're thinking. And find a way to put a positive spin on your negative thoughts.

#6. Take care of yourself

There's no doubt about it, a healthy body helps promote good mental health. Get adequate sleep. Sleep helps you tackle problems with renewed vigor. Keep physically active. Physical activity helps you burn off stress-related tension. Eat well. A balanced diet provides you with energy to handle daily stress.

#7. Enjoy a good laugh

It's healthy to spend time with people who have a positive outlook, take themselves lightly or have a sense of humor. Laughter helps reduce or relieve tension.

When you're stressed out, you may think there's nothing funny about your situation, but humor can help you cope.

Studies indicate that laughter relaxes the skeletal muscles of

Forgiveness and your health

Think of someone who's done you wrong. The wrong may be a minor insult (the jerk who nudged in front of you at the convenience store) or something extremely painful (a drunk driver who killed a loved one). What do you do when you think of that offender? Chances are you feel angry and hostile, perhaps even vengeful. Does it feel good to be in this state? Likely not, and it's not good for your health either. Feelings of anger and vengeance often cause increased blood pressure and hormone changes linked to cardiovascular disease and immune system suppression.

So what do you do?
How about try to forgive that person

Harboring vengeful and painful feelings toward someone who's hurt you puts your body under ongoing stress. In fact, a number of studies have shown heart-damaging effects from pent-up hostility. In a way, you get hurt twice — first by the actions of the other person, and then by what you do to yourself.

And what researchers have found is that people who are able to forgive — to let go of their anger and resentment — are better off both emotionally and physically.

Forgiving isn't forgetting, denying, condoning or excusing what happened. It's dropping the burden of your anger and resentment. It's refusing to let the negative feelings consume you.

The process of forgiveness often involves four phases. First, you acknowledge your pain. Next, you recognize that something has to change if you're to heal. This is followed by the hardest part — the work phase in which you strive to find a new way of thinking about the person who has harmed you. In the last phase, you begin to experience emotional relief.

If you're having difficulty letting go of your anger and hostility, consider seeking professional help.

your arms and legs, exercises your heart by raising your heart rate, and, for some, makes breathing more comfortable.

No one knows for sure why laughter has the effects it does, but one theory is that it boosts the release of endorphins, brain chemicals that create feelings of well-being.

Whatever the reason, laughter can't hurt. So, look for something to laugh about, whether it's

watching comedies or finding something humorous each day.

#8. Learn to relax

Relaxation is more than watching television or taking a break from work. True relaxation is positive and satisfying — a feeling of peace of mind. Seek out activities that give you pleasure, be it physical activity,

Turning negatives into positives

Here are some examples of typical negative mental messages and how you can give them a positive twist:

Negative thought	Positive thought
I've never done it before.	It's an opportunity to learn something new.
It's too complicated.	Let's look at it from a different angle.
I don't have the resources.	Necessity is the mother of invention.
There's not enough time.	Let's re-evaluate some priorities.
There's no way it'll work.	I can make it work.
I don't have the expertise.	I'll find people who can help me.
It's good enough.	There's always room for improvement.
It's too radical a change.	Let's take a chance.

art, music or some other hobby, and try to devote at least 30 minutes to these activities every day.

You might also experiment with relaxation techniques to help you relax when you begin to feel your muscles tightening, sense your heart rate quickening or notice the pitch of your voice rising — whatever are your warnings you're under stress.

Relaxation techniques are discussed on pages 170-172.

#9. Get professional help

You don't need to handle all of your problems alone. Help from your doctor, a mental health professional or a clergyperson

Blurred boundaries: Work vs. home life

It isn't easy to juggle the demands of a career and personal life. For most people, it's an ongoing — stressful — challenge. Part of the reason is, times have changed. Back in the '60s and '70s, most employees showed up for work Monday through Friday, worked eight to nine hours and went home to other activities. The boundaries between work and home were clear. Unfortunately, that's no longer true for many workers. Your work life may be spilling over into your personal life, blurring the line between your work and your family. Here's why:

- **Globalization of business.** Work continues around the world 24 hours a day for some people. If you work in a global organization, you might be on call 24 hours a day for troubleshooting or consulting.

- **Improvements in communication technology.** People now have the ability to work anywhere — from their home, from their car and even on vacation. And some managers expect that.

- **Longer hours.** It's not unusual for an employer to ask staff members to work longer hours than they're scheduled. For some workers, overtime may even be mandatory. If you hope to move up the career ladder, you may find yourself working more than 40 hours a week on a regular basis.

- **Changes in family roles.** Today's married worker is typically part of a dual-career couple, which can make it difficult to find time to meet commitments to children, spouse, parents, friends and home.

If you've experienced any of these challenges, you understand how easy it is for work to overtake your personal life.

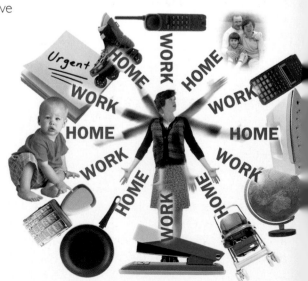

may be just what you need in order to handle stress. Many people believe seeking outside help is a sign of weakness, which adds to their sense of inadequacy, hopelessness or anger. To the contrary, it takes strength to realize that you need help and good judgment to seek it. If you need assistance finding someone who can help you, ask your doctor or employer for recommendations.

If you're experiencing physical or psychological symptoms that affect your ability to work, play or find pleasure in life, they may be a signal of something more than stress.

#10. Give yourself time

No matter what steps you take to manage stress, two simple reminders can help you be successful: practice and patience.

Practice

The steps you're taking may be new to you. In fact, at first you may feel uncomfortable doing them. Work on your coping skills daily until they come naturally. You want to get to the point where you can use them anytime, anywhere.

When you're practicing relaxation techniques, get comfortable — loosen tight clothing and remove your shoes and belt if need be.

Patience

Don't worry about how well you're doing and don't expect to see immediate benefits. It takes time and practice for stress management skills to become automatic. Keep working at it.

Is your pet helping you cope?

You may already know that the companionship and unconditional love a pet provides is priceless. But did you know that caring for a pet can bring you health benefits?

Studies show that living with a cherished animal can benefit your health in a number of ways:

- Help you cope with stress

- Lower your blood pressure

- Help you become more active

- Help you live longer after a heart attack

- Improve your mood and sense of well-being

- Make it easier to live alone

One study found that pets can buffer how you react to stress. The study compared the heart rates and blood pressure levels of people without pets and those who owned pets. People with animal companions had lower heart rates and blood pressure levels. They also had smaller increases in those levels when put under stress and faster recovery from elevated levels following stress.

In another study, stockbrokers with high blood pressure were treated with a type of medication called an angiotensin-converting enzyme (ACE) inhibitor. Of that group, those individuals who owned a pet experienced even greater reductions in blood pressure when under stress.

Studies of older adults suggest that those who shared their lives with pets were less likely to experience depression, were better able to handle living alone and were more active than their counterparts who didn't have pets.

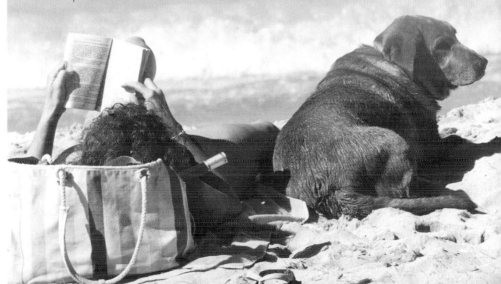

Step 9
Recharge Your Body and Mind

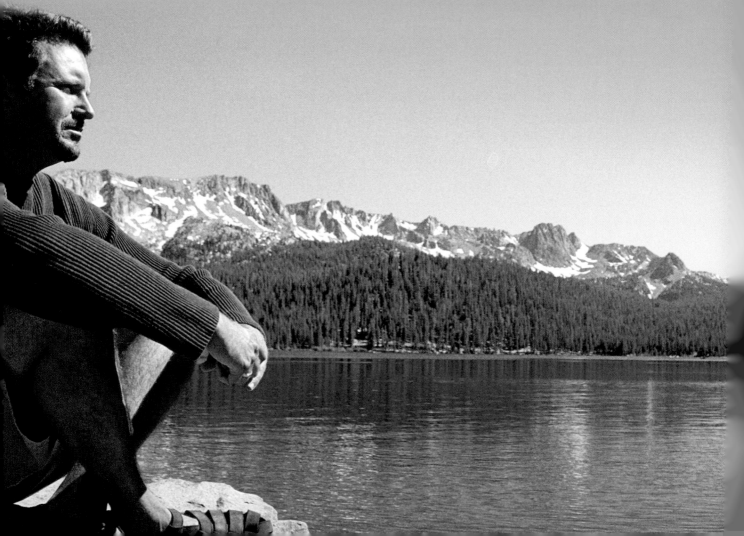

A visit with Dr. Lois Krahn

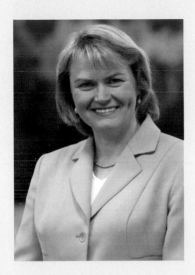

Lois Krahn, M.D.
Psychiatry & Psychology

Sleep is essential to good health. It's one of the body's basic needs. I think most people realize that if you're under stress, you don't sleep well. But I'm not sure people fully understand the deeper connections. When you don't sleep well, your ability to concentrate, to calmly deal with daily pressures, to simply feel good is compromised.

What I'm seeing more commonly, is that people are trying to get by on too little sleep. Our society has more conveniences that are available 24 hours a day, seven days a week. The Internet and e-mail are available nonstop. Stores are open longer hours, and many jobs require workers to perform shift work. There's increased temptation to get up early as well as to stay up late. The result is, more and more people aren't getting the seven to nine hours of sleep recommended by doctors.

Eventually, this behavior will catch up with you. We all know that individuals who are sleep deprived are at higher risk of accidents or performance problems because of daytime sleepiness. In addition, research indicates that people who don't get enough sleep are often at increased risk of high blood pressure, negative mood, irritability and obesity. An interesting area of ongoing research is the relationship between lack of sleep and weight gain. Individuals who get only five to six hours of sleep each night often have a harder time controlling their weight. Why is this? Are they eating to compensate for lack of sleep, or is something happening to their metabolism causing them to gain weight?

I think probably the single most important thing that people can do when it comes to good health and sleep is to make sleep a priority. People feel they need to complete all of these tasks each day and then with whatever time is leftover, sleep. We need to reverse that and set aside adequate time for sleep and then see how many of the tasks we can get done in the time remaining.

Q: Is increased caffeine consumption affecting our ability to sleep?

A: Caffeine is a very popular substance. Many people start their day with a cup of coffee, and they're correct that caffeine can improve alertness. Moderate intake of caffeine — two 8-ounce cups of coffee a day limited to the morning — is generally OK, though some people with heart conditions or high anxiety may wish to avoid caffeine. What most people don't realize is that caffeine's effects last for at least six hours. Excessive caffeine or drinking caffeine too late in the day can cause problems, including trouble sleeping at night. You also shouldn't use caffeine to replace sleep.

Q: How do I know if my snoring is associated with sleep apnea?

A: Snoring may occur only under certain circumstances, such as having a glass of wine or lying on your back. In these cases, snoring usually isn't cause for concern. However, any snoring is an indication that the upper airway is narrow enough that the surrounding tissue vibrates. If your snoring is loud and continuous, regardless of body position, this is more worrisome. It can be a warning of a potentially serious sleep disorder. Seek medical attention if your snoring is accompanied by pauses in breathing, awakenings at night, daytime sleepiness or elevated blood pressure. These features are all suggestive of obstructive sleep apnea, a condition that interrupts breathing while you sleep.

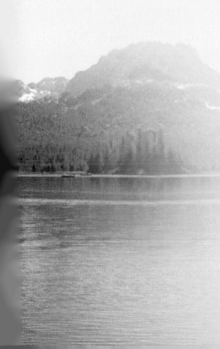

Give yourself a break

Rest and relaxation are basic necessities. They're as fundamental to your health as fresh air, nutritious food and physical activity. The problem is — most people don't get enough.

You may think that taking a few minutes to unwind at the end of the day is all of the relaxation you need. Unfortunately, a few minutes don't provide the health benefits of deep relaxation. When you truly relax, you eliminate unhealthy tension from your body and mind.

And when it comes to sleep, one study after another indicates that most Americans are coming up short. Lack of sleep affects not only your energy level but also your mental and social functioning. Too little sleep can make it more difficult for you to concentrate, and you may be impatient with others, less interactive in your relationships and less productive at work.

More importantly, too little sleep can be downright dangerous. According to the National Highway Traffic Safety Administration, more than 100,000 automobile crashes each year are the result of drivers falling asleep at the wheel.

Your body needs downtime

With so many things to do each day, it's easy to put off time for yourself. But it's important that you take time a few days a week, if not every day, to relax.

Want a good reason why? We'll give you several. Relaxation:

- Slows your heart rate, meaning less work for your heart
- Reduces your blood pressure
- Increases blood flow to your major muscles
- Slows your breathing rate
- Lessens muscle tension
- Reduces signs and symptoms of illness, such as headaches, nausea, diarrhea and pain
- Lessens unhealthy emotional responses such as anger, crying, anxiety, apprehension and frustration
- Gives you more energy
- Improves your concentration

Learning to relax

So how do you truly relax? Use relaxation skills — they aren't as difficult as they may seem. More than skill, relaxation takes patience and practice. Don't be discouraged if you don't feel the benefits right away. They'll come.

Following are some techniques you can use to calm your mind and body. You don't need to do them all. Just choose one or two that you feel would work best for you.

Relaxed breathing

This form of relaxation focuses on deep, relaxed breathing as a way to relieve tension and stress. Rehearse it throughout the day so that it becomes natural and you can apply it when needed.

Before you begin, find a comfortable position. Lie on a bed or couch, or sit on a chair. Then do the following:

- **Inhale.** With your mouth closed and your shoulders relaxed, inhale slowly and deeply through your nose to the count of six. Allow the air to fill your lungs, pushing your abdomen out.
- **Pause** for a second.
- **Exhale.** Slowly release air through your mouth as you count to six.
- **Pause** for a second.
- **Repeat.** Complete this breathing cycle several times.

Progressive muscle relaxation

Progressive muscle relaxation is a stress-reducing technique that involves relaxing a series of muscles one at a time.

Begin by sitting or lying in a comfortable position. Loosen tight clothing and close your eyes. Mentally scan your body, beginning with your face and working downward. The goal is to tense each muscle group for five seconds, then relax for at least 30 seconds. Repeat once before moving to the next muscle group.

- **Upper face.** Lift your eyebrows to the ceiling, feeling the tension in your forehead.
- **Central face.** Squint your eyes and wrinkle your nose and mouth, feeling the tension in the center of your face.
- **Lower face.** Clench your teeth and pull back the cor-

ners of your mouth toward your ears.

- **Neck**. Gently touch your chin to your chest. Feel the pull in the back of your neck.
- **Shoulders**. Pull your shoulders up toward your ears, feeling the tension in your shoulders, head, neck and upper back.
- **Upper arms**. Pull your arms back and press your elbows toward the sides of your body. Try not to tense your lower arms. Feel the tension in your upper arms, shoulders and back.
- **Hands and lower arms.** Make a fist and pull up your wrists. Feel the tension in your hands and lower arms.
- **Chest, shoulders and upper back**. Pull your shoulders back as if trying to make your shoulder blades touch.
- **Stomach**. Pull your stomach toward your spine, tightening your abdominal muscles.
- **Upper legs**. Squeeze your knees together. Feel the tension in your thighs.
- **Lower legs**. Bend your ankles so that your toes point toward your face. Feel the tension in your calves.
- **Feet**. Turn your feet inward and curl your toes up and out.

Meditation

Another way to relax is to use meditation techniques to calm your body and ease your mind. Meditation helps you enter a deeply restful state. As you begin to relax, your breathing slows, your heart rate decreases and tension in your muscles lessens.

How to meditate

You don't have to twist your legs into a pretzel to learn how to meditate. All you need is to find a quiet place where you won't be disturbed. Sit or lie in a comfortable position and determine a focus for your mind:

- **Focus on your breath.** Breathe through your nose and pay attention to some aspect of your breathing, such as the pause between breaths or the sensation of air leaving your nose.
- **Focus on a word, phrase or prayer.** In Transcendental Meditation you mentally repeat a word or sound assigned by your instructor, called a mantra. But you can choose your own mantra, or you can count from one to four over and over. You can also coordinate your mantra with your breathing.
- **Focus on the moment.** This form of meditation is also known as mindfulness meditation. You become aware of sensations, sounds and thoughts. You simply notice them and let them go. Or you may notice the sensations in your body — stomach growling or thigh cramping.

Many people meditate with their eyes closed. Others prefer to keep their eyes partially open with a soft focus. It doesn't matter whether you lie down or sit on the floor, a chair or a meditation cushion, as long as you're comfortable. But don't get so comfortable that you fall asleep.

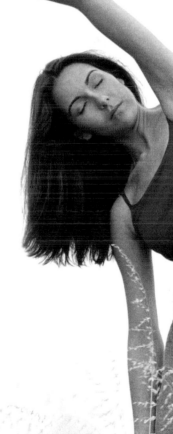

During meditation, you sit still and make an effort to focus on one single thing, such as a particular image or word or phrase. When your thoughts wander — as they inevitably do — you bring your focus back to where it was.

Meditation can reduce your body's response to the hormones it produces when you're stressed, such as the hormone adrenaline. Adrenaline can raise your blood pressure and make your blood more likely to clot — both risk factors for heart disease.

There are many different forms of meditation. You may want to take a class to help you get started. Begin with a five-minute session once or twice a day and, if you can, try to work up to 20-minute sessions.

Visualization

Also known as guided imagery, visualization involves lying quietly and picturing yourself in a pleasant and peaceful setting.

- **Allow thoughts to flow through your mind.** But don't focus on any of them. Tell yourself that you're relaxed and calm, that your hands are heavy and warm — or cool if you're hot — that your heart is beating calmly.
- **Breathe slowly.** And breathe regularly and deeply.
- **Think of a calming setting.** Once you're relaxed, imagine yourself in a favorite place.
- **Let go.** After five or 10 minutes, rouse yourself gradually.

Brain studies of people undergoing visualization indicate that picturing a certain setting stimulates the same parts of your brain that are stimulated during the actual experience. If sitting by the ocean relaxes you, you may achieve the same level of relaxation with visualization as if you were actually there.

Yoga

Yoga is an ancient practice that aims to induce physical, mental and spiritual well-being through a combination of postures (asanas), breathing techniques and meditation. This practice is increasingly popular among people seeking relaxation or a spiritual path, or trying to improve their flexibility, coordination, balance, strength and endurance.

According to the National Center for Complementary and Alternative Medicine, the benefits of yoga — when practiced regularly — may include reduced anxiety, slowed breathing, lowered blood pressure, altered brain waves and more efficient blood flow. Many yoga enthusiasts claim that yoga can treat specific mental and physical disorders, but there aren't enough randomized, controlled studies to support the claims.

Make sure to find an experienced instructor who adapts the postures to your levels of flexibility. At the very least, yoga can relax you, and some forms may improve your physical conditioning. But yoga isn't easy. It requires discipline and concentration.

Tai chi

Tai chi is sometimes described as "meditation in motion." This ancient Chinese form of exercise involves slow, gentle, dance-like movements. Tai chi helps relieve overall stress and increases feelings of well-being. It also offers physical benefits. Tai chi helps relax and strengthen muscles and joints to improve stability, coordination and balance.

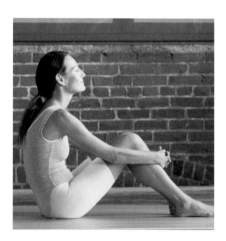

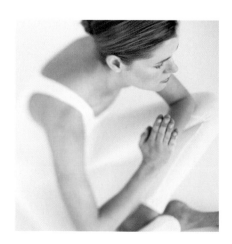

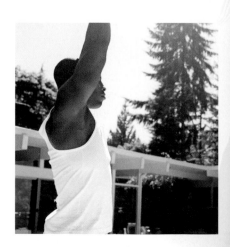

Save time for sleep

So how much sleep is enough? The amount needed each night varies from person to person. The average is seven and a half to eight hours of sleep a night, but some people feel fine with only four to six hours while others need up to nine hours. More important than counting hours is assessing how you feel during the day. If you feel alert, are functioning well and aren't tired, even when you relax for a few minutes, you're probably getting enough sleep.

But many Americans don't get the sleep they need. More than 100 million Americans of all ages have occasional sleep problems. For many people, a hectic lifestyle and increased work demands put time at a premium, and sleep often takes a back seat.

Despite the popular notion that you need less sleep as you age, sleep needs generally remain constant throughout adulthood. The amount of sleep your body and brain require changes little.

Not all sleep is the same

There are two types of sleep — non-rapid eye movement (NREM) and rapid eye movement (REM).

NREM sleep

Your nightly journey begins as you pass into stage 1 of NREM sleep, a light sleep. During NREM sleep, your brain activity and body functions slow. This type of sleep has three other stages: Stage 2 is the one in which you spend the most time. During this stage, your brain waves become larger, with bursts of electrical activity. Stages 3 and 4, called deep sleep, are the most restful. In these stages, brain waves are large and slow, and you're more difficult to awaken.

REM sleep

REM, or dream, sleep occurs about one and a half to two hours after you fall asleep. During REM sleep, your eyes move rapidly behind your closed lids, hence the name. This is a period of greater activity during which you dream and your body functions speed up.

During REM sleep, your brain waves show faster electrical activity at lower amplitude than at other sleep stages, a pattern that's similar to the brain waves of wakefulness. This suggests that you do more thinking, in the form of dreaming, in this state than in the other sleep stages. People awakened during REM sleep may recall vivid dreams.

Throughout the night, you continually move from one stage of sleep to another in cycles that can last from 70 to 90 minutes each.

Are you running low?

Many people think they're getting adequate sleep but really aren't. You may not be getting the right amount and quality of sleep if:

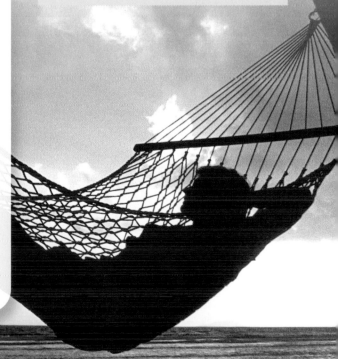

- You routinely ignore your alarm clock or snatch a few extra minutes to snooze before getting up
- You look forward to catching up on your sleep on the weekends
- You have to fight to stay awake during long meetings, in overheated rooms or after a heavy meal
- You're irritable with co-workers, family and friends
- You have difficulty concentrating or remembering
- You wake repeatedly throughout the night
- You wake up groggy and not feeling refreshed
- Your spouse or partner complains about your snoring or fitful sleeping

To nap or not to nap?

It's midafternoon and your eyelids are getting heavy. You try to ignore the feeling, but you have to fight to stay awake. Should you follow the irresistible urge to snooze, or will that keep you from sleeping well at night?

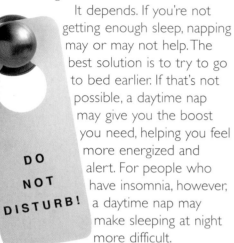

It depends. If you're not getting enough sleep, napping may or may not help. The best solution is to try to go to bed earlier. If that's not possible, a daytime nap may give you the boost you need, helping you feel more energized and alert. For people who have insomnia, however, a daytime nap may make sleeping at night more difficult.

An urge for a midday nap is built into your body's biological clock. Usually between 1 p.m. and 4 p.m., you experience a slight drop in your body temperature, indicating nap time. Most Americans ignore the urge, but people of many other cultures incorporate it into their lifestyles.

To discover how naps affect your energy level and the quality of your nighttime sleep, do an experiment. Take a daily nap for a week. The next week, don't nap. Every morning, rank your sleep quality on a 10-point scale. Every evening, rate your day on a similar scale. After two weeks, judge whether naps work for you.

If you do nap, keep it short — limit it to 20 or 30 minutes late in the morning or in the midafternoon. And don't rely on naps to keep you going. Try to get enough sleep at night to avoid compiling a sleep deficit.

Tips for better sleep

Sleeping patterns are highly individual, and techniques that help one person sleep better may not help someone else. The first steps to take if you have trouble sleeping, are simple changes in your daily and bedtime routines. Here are some suggestions that may improve your sleep:

- **Stick to a sleep schedule.** Go to bed and get up at about the same time every day, including weekends. Limit your time in bed to no more than eight hours. Too much time in bed can disrupt sleep.

- **Establish and follow a bedtime ritual.** In the evening, slow the pace of your activities before bedtime.

- **Exercise and stay active.** Aim for 30 minutes of moderately vigorous exercise most days of the week. Physical activity enhances deep, refreshing sleep. But avoid exercising too close to bedtime. Afternoon exercise seems to have the most positive effect on sleep.

- **Don't eat or drink a lot before bedtime.** A light snack may help you sleep, but avoid heavy meals and fluids or foods that stimulate stomach acid production, which can cause heartburn. Drink less liquid before bedtime so that you don't have to get up at night to go to the bathroom.

- **Avoid or limit caffeine, nicotine and alcohol.** Don't drink caffeinated coffee, tea, cocoa or cola after your noon meal. Don't smoke before bedtime because nicotine can cause shallow sleeping and sleeplessness.

- **Schedule worry time.** If worries keep you awake, attempt to deal with them before you go to bed. Set aside a "worry time" during the day. Make a list of problems and identify possible solutions.

- **Find ways to relax.** Taking a warm bath or drinking a warm decaffeinated beverage may help. Or you can try relaxation exercises.

- **Create a comfortable sleep environment.** Keep your bedroom quiet, dark and comfortably cool. Your bed should be comfortable.

- **Don't watch the clock.** If a bedside clock keeps you awake at night, put it in a dresser drawer or under the bed.

- **Don't rely on sleeping pills.** If you do take a sleep medication for a few days, reduce the dosage gradually when you want to discontinue using it.

- **Check your medications.** Ask your doctor if your medications may be contributing to your insomnia. Check the label of over-the-counter products to see if they contain caffeine or other stimulants, such as ephedrine or pseudoephedrine.

- **If sleep doesn't come naturally, read a book, listen to music or watch television until you feel drowsy.** But don't sleep later in the morning. Keep a firm time for going to bed and waking up.

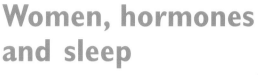

Women, hormones and sleep

Menstruation, pregnancy and menopause all can affect how well women sleep. That's because changing levels of the female sex hormones estrogen and progesterone influence the quality of your sleep.

During your menstrual cycle, the hormone progesterone rises after ovulation and may cause you to feel more sleepy or tired. Progesterone levels peak around days 19 to 21 of the cycle and then begin to fall. During this low point, you may find it more difficult to fall asleep. During the week before menstruation, some women who experience premenstrual syndrome (PMS) commonly report insomnia followed by daytime sleepiness. Sleep disturbances during pregnancy also are common, especially as the pregnancy progresses.

It's during menopause, though, that women generally experience the greatest difficulty with sleep. Changing and decreasing levels of the hormone estrogen can cause symptoms that disrupt sleep, such as hot flashes. Snoring also is more common and more severe in postmenopausal women. Sleep apnea — a condition in which your airway is repeatedly obstructed while you sleep, interfering with breathing — is less common in women than in men. However, once women reach menopause, they generally develop sleep apnea at about the same rate as do men.

Overcome insomnia

In addition to hectic schedules and busy workdays, various sleep disorders can deprive people of their needed slumber. Insomnia, characterized by difficulty falling or staying asleep, is the most common sleep problem.

Insomnia is defined as an inability to get enough sleep, to the point where your daytime functioning is affected. Almost everyone has occasional sleepless nights, perhaps due to stress, heartburn or drinking too much caffeine or alcohol. Insomnia differs in that it occurs on a regular or frequent basis.

About one-third of all people experience insomnia at some point. The condition can be temporary or chronic.

Causes

The causes of insomnia are many and varied. They include:

Stress and anxiety

Concerns about work, school, health or family can keep your mind too active and unable to relax for sleep. Excessive boredom, such as during a long illness, also can create stress and keep you awake. Everyday anxieties as well as severe anxiety disorders may keep your mind too alert to sleep.

Depression

Often, people who are depressed either sleep too much or have trouble falling asleep. This may be due to chemical imbalances in the brain or because anxiety that can accompany depression prevents relaxation.

Environment or work changes

Long-distance air travel or having to work a late or early shift can disrupt your body's circadian rhythms, which help control sleep.

Age

Insomnia becomes more prevalent with age.

Stimulants and medications

Drinking coffee, tea or colas can trigger insomnia. If you're especially sensitive to caffeine, even a cup or two during the day can keep you awake at night. Smoking also can contribute to insomnia. Nicotine is an addictive stimulant that can keep you awake. In addition, smokers may experience withdrawal symptoms at night, making it more difficult both to fall asleep at night and to wake up in the morning.

Do you have insomnia?

Signs and symptoms of insomnia include the following:

- Difficulty falling asleep at night
- Frequent awakenings during the night
- Waking up too early in the morning
- Daytime fatigue or sleepiness
- Daytime irritability

Less sleep, less sex

Approximately one-fourth of respondents to a 2005 poll on sleep habits reported having sex less often or losing interest in sex because they were too tired.

The poll, conducted by the National Sleep Foundation, found that about 75 percent of adults frequently have trouble sleeping, such as not being able to fall asleep, waking during the night or snoring.

In addition to poorer health, lower productivity on the job and greater danger on the roads, it appears that lack of sleep also equates to a less vibrant sex life.

Some prescription medications, including steroids, antidepressants and some high blood pressure medications, can interfere with sleep. Many over-the-counter medications, including some brands of aspirin, decongestants and weight-loss products, contain caffeine and other stimulants. Antihistamines may initially make you groggy, but they can worsen urinary problems, causing you to get up more often at night.

Alcohol

Although a drink or two of an alcoholic beverage seems to help some people relax enough to fall asleep, even moderate amounts of alcohol can distort normal sleeping patterns. Alcohol may help you get to sleep, but it also frequently wakes you up in the middle of the night.

Learned insomnia

After a few nights of poor sleep, you may start worrying about being able to sleep. The more you worry, the less you sleep. You may come to associate being in your bedroom with being awake. Most people with this condition sleep better when they're away from their usual sleep environment or when they're not trying to sleep, such as when they're watching television.

Illnesses and life changes

Diseases or disorders that cause pain — conditions such as arthritis, fibromyalgia or a nerve disorder (neuropathy) — can interfere with sleep. A number of other conditions, such as allergies or thyroid problems, can disrupt your sleep. Conditions that occur with age, such as menopause, also may interfere with sleep.

Is it more than just insomnia?

Sometimes, what appears to be insomnia may actually be something else, or your insomnia may be masking another condition.

Depression

Depression and insomnia can produce similar symptoms, and the two conditions often occur together.

Disruptive sleep patterns, which are a common symptom of depression, are one of the leading causes of insomnia. On the other hand, insomnia's impact on mood, productivity and well-being can lead to depression.

Some people who visit a doctor for insomnia don't realize that they're experiencing depression. Therefore, don't be surprised if your doctor asks you questions about your moods and lifestyle to determine if you might be depressed.

Not surprisingly, early treatment of insomnia may reduce your risk of developing depression, and treating depression often solves the problem of insomnia.

Anxiety

Excessive anxiety and anxiety disorders also can produce insomnia.

Often, insomnia caused by anxiety or tension begins during, or shortly after, a stressful period in your life. It may be helpful to think about when your insomnia began to see if you can link the condition with a life change or some type of stress or persistent worry.

Medications, as well as relaxation techniques, are often helpful in treating anxiety-induced insomnia.

Medications to help you sleep

It's an easy way to improve sleep — just take a pill. But not all products promising to help you sleep better are effective, or good for you.

Prescription sleeping pills

If you're having trouble sleeping, your doctor may prescribe a sleeping pill until other steps to improve your sleep — such as reducing stress or increasing physical activity — have time to work. Sleeping pills aren't recommended for long-term use because they can lead to dependence and other unwanted side effects.

Benzodiazepines are older forms of sleeping pills. They include medications such as flurazepam (Dalmane) and estazolam (ProSom), which slow your central nervous system. After four to six months of use, they not only lose their effectiveness but also disturb your sleep patterns and contribute to insomnia.

Newer sleeping pills such as eszopiclone (Lunesta) zolpidem (Ambien) and zaleplon (Sonata) are less habit-forming than the previous ones, but they're still not recommended for long-term use.

Your doctor may caution you against taking sleeping pills if you drink alcohol or have to operate machinery soon after waking up. Alcohol, which also is a sedative, should be avoided because it exaggerates the effects of sleep medications.

Antidepressants

Treating depression can help improve sleep, but most antidepressant medications don't work right away, and some can even interfere with sleep.

Your doctor may prescribe a low dose of a sedating antidepressant medication, such as trazodone (Desyrel), nortriptyline (Aventyl, Pamelor) or amitriptyline, to help you sleep. Sedating antidepressants taken in low doses aren't habit-forming, and they can be taken for a longer period than can other sleep medications.

Over-the-counter sleeping pills

Over-the-counter products are less effective than are prescription medications. Many over-the-counter sleep products contain antihistamines to induce drowsiness. These products are OK for occasional sleepless nights, but they, too, often lose their effectiveness the more you take them. Many nonprescription products also contain diphenhydramine, which can cause difficulty urinating and may make you feel drowsy during the daytime.

Melatonin is an over-the-counter product marketed to help prevent jet lag and overcome insomnia, among other things. Melatonin is a hormone that occurs naturally in the human body and helps establish your sleep-wake cycle. The supplements sold in stores are synthetic or animal forms of the hormone. Only about 5 percent of people who've taken the supplements report better sleep.

The herbal supplement valerian has been shown to help some people fall asleep more quickly and improve sleep quality. As with melatonin, its effectiveness varies and more study is needed.

Some people find drinking chamomile tea before bedtime to be helpful.

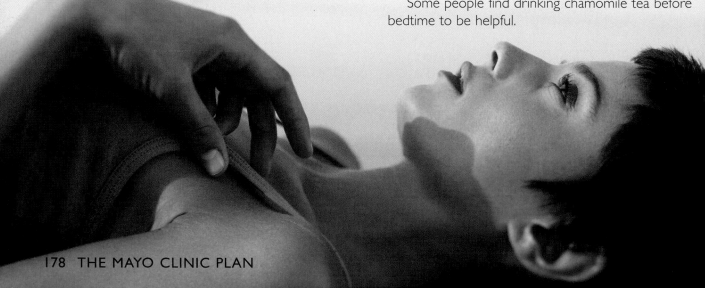

Eating too much too late

Eating too much before going to bed may cause you to feel physically uncomfortable when you lie down, making it difficult to sleep. After overeating, many people experience heartburn, a reflux of food from the stomach into the esophagus. This uncomfortable feeling may keep you awake.

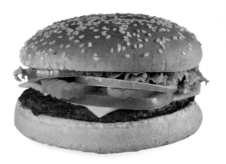

Poor sleep environment

A bed partner's snoring, a barking dog and a room that's too hot are just a few of the environmental conditions that can make it difficult to get to sleep.

Treating insomnia

Insomnia is usually temporary, and often self-help measures — simple changes in your daily routine — can treat the condition. If self-help measures don't work, your doctor may recommend other approaches.

Relaxation training

Relaxation training in which you learn different ways to relax your body and mind can be helpful if you're having difficulty sleeping due to stress or anxiety.

Stimulus control

Stimulus control teaches you to associate your bedroom with sleep. You may be asked to limit activities in your bedroom to sleep and sex, to go to bed only when you're sleepy and to leave the bedroom if you don't fall asleep quickly.

Sleep restriction

Your doctor may ask you to reduce the time you spend in bed to as few as five hours a night, then gradually increase that amount of time until you reach your desired quality and duration of sleep. The idea is to reduce the amount of time you spend in bed without sleeping. Nine out of 10 people with insomnia stay in bed longer than necessary.

Medication

To help you sleep, your doctor may prescribe medication. Often, though, sleep medications are only a short-term treatment until other therapies begin to work.

Snoring

Snoring is very common. Approximately half of men and one-third of women — most age 50 or older — snore. But snoring isn't reserved just for "old folks." It affects younger adults, too. Snoring occurs when air flows past tissues in your throat that are relaxed. The air causes the tissues to vibrate. You hear this vibration as snoring.

If snoring is disturbing your sleep, you could have a condition called sleep apnea, and a sleep study may be necessary. Even if your snoring isn't associated with sleep apnea, it can be disruptive to your partner's sleep. And research has shown that snoring may disrupt your sleep as well — even though you may not realize it — making you sleepy during the day. Evidence also suggests that loud, frequent snoring may lead to high blood pressure.

Treatment of snoring is much the same as that of sleep apnea. Losing weight, sleeping on your side, treating nasal congestion, and avoiding alcohol and sedating medications may help.

Nasal strips help many people increase the area of their nasal passages, enhancing their breathing. Surgery also is sometimes performed. It isn't advised for occasional or light snoring, but may be an option if your snoring is frequent, loud and disruptive.

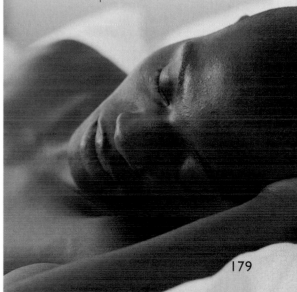

Step 10
Play It Safe

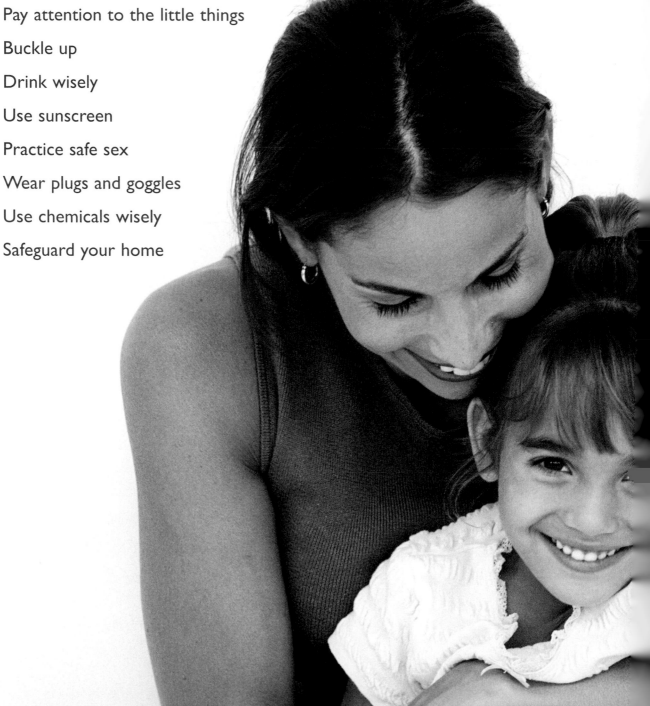

Most of us don't pay enough attention to safety issues. Unintentional injuries are the leading cause of death in the United States for people under age 35, and the fifth-leading cause of death overall. You make safety-related decisions all day long — whether to buckle up, wear safety glasses and earplugs, or follow safety directions on labels. The goal of safer living is lowering your risk of an injury. This doesn't mean you have to live in a bubble and be insulated from all that's fun and interesting in the world. It means taking five seconds of extra effort to better protect yourself.

Unless you have a background in statistics, knowing what your greatest safety risks are can be difficult. Yet, it's really important. Let me give you an example. The risk of dying of a lightning strike is less than one in a million. The risk of dying in a motor vehicle accident is about one in 7,000. In a thunderstorm, nearly everyone would take steps to avoid getting struck by lightning — going indoors or avoiding tall trees or open areas. But, not everyone will buckle up their seat belts.

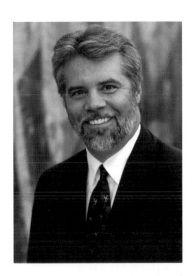

Philip Hagen, M.D.
Preventive Medicine

Q: What safety issue concerns you the most?

A: Motor vehicle safety is still the biggest safety issue we face. We've made huge strides in the last 30 years in making cars safer, making roads safer and encouraging the use of seat belts. Still, more than 40,000 people die each year in motor vehicle accidents. Reducing your risk of an automobile accident is relatively simple — always wear seat belts, don't drink and drive, and avoid distractions such as eating and talking on the phone.

Here are the top five safety-related causes of death in the United States in 2002 (the latest figures available):

• Motor vehicle accidents: 44,065 deaths

• Firearm-related: 30,242 deaths

• Poisoning: 26,435 deaths

• Falls: 17,116 deaths

• Suffocation: 12,791 deaths

Another leading cause of death — especially among younger people — is suicide. We think most suicides are preventable.

Q: What advice do you give parents?

A: One way to practice safety is to be prepared. I'll give you an example. A colleague of mine had just read information on the Heimlich maneuver. A week later, one of her children choked on some food. She successfully stepped in and saved the child. It's a dramatic example, but part of being safe is being prepared. Unsafe situations are often unpredictable — knowing how to react can be lifesaving. Taking a Red Cross first-aid course and making sure your kids receive swimming lessons at an early age are just two examples of being prepared. Another example is a periodic review of what to do if a child ingests something toxic.

Pay attention to the little things

As you go about making healthy changes in your life, don't forget the common-sense stuff. We're talking here about good health basics — wearing your seat belt, putting on sunscreen, not driving after you've been drinking alcohol, making sure your home is equipped with working smoke detectors, and so forth.

You can do everything possible to keep fit — exercise, eat well, see your doctor — but if you don't also pay attention to basic safety precautions, all of your effort may be for naught.

Did you know?

- More than 16,000 individuals killed in automobile accidents in 2003 (the latest figures available) and approximately 250,000 individuals injured weren't wearing seat belts.

- In 45 percent of motorcycle deaths in 2003, the victim wasn't wearing a helmet.

- Nearly 70 percent of fatal bicycle crashes involve head injuries, but only about 20 percent to 25 percent of bicyclists wear helmets.

- Universal helmet use by children ages 4 to 15 would prevent up to 49,000 head injuries and 55,000 face and scalp injuries each year.

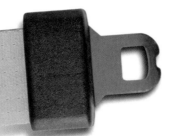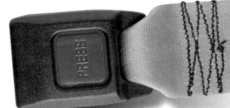

Buckle up

The snap of a buckle means a lot when it comes to your health.

In the car

Approximately 45,000 people die on the nation's roads and highways every year. Many more individuals are severely injured. This terrible toll is often the result of alcohol or carelessness. To help ensure your safety:

Always wear a seat belt

Seat belts save lives. Wear one every time you get into a car, even if you're traveling only a short distance. Most accidents occur within a few miles of home. Make sure that your passengers wear seat belts, too.

Place children in car seats or booster seats

Always buckle up your child when traveling by car. In most states, children who weigh less than 40 pounds must ride in specially designed car seats. And in some states, children must ride in booster seats until they reach a size where an adult seat belt will fit them properly.

On the street

Three of four cyclists killed in cycle-related accidents die of head injuries. That's why it's important that you always wear a helmet. A Mayo Clinic study found that children are more likely to wear helmets if their parents do.

Your helmet should fit well, have a durable outer shell and a polystyrene liner. Adjustable foam pads help ensure a proper fit in the front, back and sides.

On the water

When operating a boat or personal watercraft, always wear a lifejacket, or personal flotation device (PFD). Even if you're a good swimmer, you should wear a life jacket in case you get knocked unconscious or injured in an accident.

Road hazards

Automobile accidents are often the result of inattention. To reduce your risk of an accident:

Avoid distractions
Control the behavior of children in your car. Don't let the radio, your cell phone, an interesting conversation or a roadside attraction distract you from your driving.

Check medications
We all know that alcohol and automobiles are a deadly combination. It's also important that you don't get behind the wheel if you've taken medications that make you drowsy. Sedating medications impair your reaction time and can cause you to fall asleep.

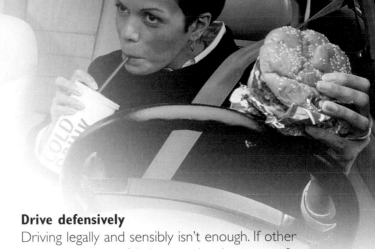

Drive defensively
Driving legally and sensibly isn't enough. If other drivers aren't careful, they can be the cause of an accident. Never assume that other drivers will drive responsibly. Driving defensively means that you're aware of other vehicles at all times and are prepared to take evasive action.

Drink wisely

For every news story you read about the benefits of alcohol, another seems to warn you of the risks. The conflicting information can be confusing and frustrating.

Though it's unclear whether alcohol's health benefits outweigh its risks, what is certain is that anything more than moderate drinking can negate any benefits alcohol may provide.

What's moderate drinking? Two drinks a day if you're a man younger than age 65 or one drink a day if you're a man 65 and older or a woman.

So, is it OK to enjoy a glass of wine with dinner or a bottle of beer during an evening with friends? Yes, provided you limit the amount and alcohol doesn't exacerbate an existing health problem or interfere with medications you take.

If you don't currently drink alcohol, should you start doing so to take advantage of its potential health benefits? Most doctors will say no. You likely have good reasons for not consuming alcohol, and there are other ways that you can reduce your risk of health problems.

The pros
Evidence suggests that moderate alcohol use may:
* Reduce your risk of dying of a heart attack
* Reduce your risk of strokes
* Lower your risk of gallstones
* Possibly reduce your risk of diabetes

The cons
Excess alcohol consumption can lead to a number of serious health problems, including:

* Cancer of the mouth, pharynx, larynx, esophagus, liver and breast
* High blood pressure, heart failure and stroke
* Elevated levels of triglycerides in the blood
* Alcoholic cirrhosis of the liver
* Chronic pancreatitis
* Miscarriage
* Fetal alcohol syndrome in an unborn child, including slow growth and nervous system problems

Who shouldn't drink alcohol?
People with certain health conditions shouldn't drink alcohol at all, since even small amounts could cause problems. It's best not to drink alcohol if you have:

- Had a hemorrhagic stroke
- Liver or pancreatic disease
- Been diagnosed with precancerous changes of the esophagus, larynx, pharynx or mouth

If you have a family history of alcoholism, be particularly cautious when it comes to drinking alcohol, as you may be at higher risk of alcoholism.

Also be careful if you take medications regularly. Discuss your medications — both prescription and over-the-counter products — and the potential for alcohol interactions with your doctor or a pharmacist.

Examples of some medications that can interact with alcohol include antibiotics, antidepressants, anti-seizure medications, pain relievers, antihistamines and sleeping pills.

Use sunscreen

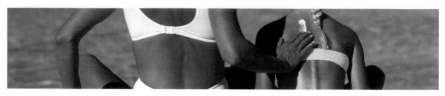

Skin cancer is the most common form of cancer. Doctors diagnose skin cancer in more than 1 million Americans each year. The heartening news about this cancer is that it can be prevented. There are many things you can do to reduce your risk of skin cancer. One of the easiest is simply to wear sunscreen.

Sunscreens don't filter out all harmful ultraviolet (UV) radiation from the sun — especially the radiation that can lead to melanoma, the most serious form of skin cancer — but they do play a major role in providing sun protection.

Wear sunscreen both in the summer and in the winter when you're outside. For the most protection, apply sunscreen 30 minutes before sun exposure and reapply it every two hours throughout the day. Also be sure to reapply it after swimming or exercising. Apply sunscreen to young children before they go outdoors, and teach older children how to use sunscreen to protect themselves.

Keep sunscreen in your car as well as with your gardening tools and sports and camping gear to remind yourself and your family to use it.

Most people use sunscreens too sparingly. Labels on most sunscreens call for liberal and frequent applications. A liberal application is 1 ounce — equal to about 2 tablespoons. That's how much you need to cover all exposed parts of the body.

Are you sunscreen savvy?

Not all sunscreens are the same. Be sure to use a broad-spectrum sunscreen with a sun protection factor (SPF) of at least 15. Broad-spectrum products provide protection against both UVA and UVB radiation. Use sunscreen on all exposed skin, including your

Matters of the heart

Some of the greatest potential benefits from alcohol appear to be heart-related. Studies show that one or two drinks a day may reduce your risk of coronary artery disease — damage to the arteries that lead to your heart. A large U.S. survey spanning 15 years found the incidence of coronary artery disease was lower in men who drank alcohol than in men who didn't.

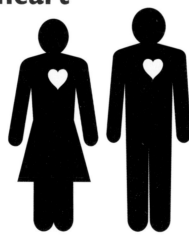

Another study found that men who consumed two drinks or less at least three times a week were about one-third less likely to have a heart attack than were men who didn't drink.

Keep in mind that studies involving alcohol's impact on health so far have been observational — meaning there's still a lot we don't know and more study is needed.

Other ways to shield your skin

Sunscreen isn't the only way to protect yourself against the sun. To reduce your risk of cancer, follow these simple precautions:

- **Don't use products touted as tan accelerators, such as coconut, cocoa or baby oil.** These products don't make you tan faster, and they don't protect you from ultraviolet (UV) radiation.

- **Try to avoid the sun between 10 a.m. and 3 p.m.** The sun's rays are strongest during this period, even in winter or when the sky is cloudy, so try to schedule outdoor activities for other times of the day. Remember that you absorb UV radiation year-round, and clouds offer little protection from damaging UV rays.

- **Wear protective clothing.** Sunscreens don't provide complete protection from UV rays. That's why it's a good idea to also wear dark, tightly woven clothing that covers your arms and legs, and a broad-brimmed hat, which provides more protection than a base-ball cap or visor. Some companies also design photoprotective clothing. Your dermatologist can recommend an appropriate brand. Don't forget sunglasses. Look for those that block out both UVA and UVB rays.

- **Avoid tanning beds and tan-accelerating agents.** Tanning beds emit UVA rays, which may be as dangerous as UVB rays, especially since UVA light penetrates deeper into your skin and causes pre-cancerous skin lesions.

- **Be aware of sun-sensitizing medications.** Some common prescription and over-the-counter drugs — including antibiotics; certain cholesterol, high blood pressure and diabetes medications; birth control pills; nonsteroidal anti-inflammatory drugs such as ibuprofen (Advil, Motrin, others); and the acne medication isotretinoin (Accutane) — can make your skin more sensitive to sunlight. If you take a medication that increases sun sensitivity, be sure to take extra precautions.

- **Have regular skin examinations.** If you're older than age 40, talk to your doctor about periodic skin examinations. If you're at high risk of developing melanoma, discuss how often to have an exam.

- **Check your skin regularly, and report any changes to your doctor.** Examine your skin often for new skin growths or changes in existing moles, freckles, bumps and birthmarks. With the help of a mirror, check the back of your neck and ears, your back, and the back or your arms and legs.

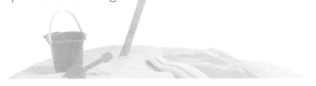

The ABCDs of melanoma

Melanoma is often curable if you find it early. Follow this self-examination guide, adapted from the American Academy of Dermatology's A-B-C-D guide, to determine if an unusual mole or suspicious spot on your skin may be melanoma.

A is for asymmetry
Symmetrical round or oval growths are usually noncancerous (benign). Look for irregular shapes where one half is a different shape than the other half.

B is for border
Growths with irregular, notched, scalloped or vaguely defined borders need to be examined.

C is for color
Look for growths that have many colors or an uneven distribution of color. Often, growths that are the same color all over are benign.

D is for diameter
Have your doctor check any growths that are larger than 6 millimeters, about the diameter of a pencil eraser.

lips, the tops of your ears, and the backs of your hands and neck.

Most sunscreens provide physical protection, chemical protection or a combination of both. Knowing the difference can help you select the best product for you and your family.

Physical sunscreens contain ingredients such as zinc oxide and titanium dioxide. These form an opaque film that reflects UV rays before they can penetrate your skin. Chemical sunscreens, on the other hand, absorb sunlight before it can cause any damage. Combination products do a little of both.

Improved labeling

Sunscreen labels can be confusing, and sometimes they are misleading. That's why the Food and Drug Administration has instituted new labeling guidelines.

- Certain words can no longer be used, such as the terms *sun block* (no product actually blocks all UV rays), *all-day* (no sunscreen lasts all day) and *waterproof* (all sunscreens wash off in water to some extent). The new term is *water-resistant*.
- Sunscreens claiming an SPF higher than 30 are now labeled 30+, rather than 45 or 60, because tests show little difference among products with SPF factors above 30.
- Products that don't contain sunscreen are required by law to clearly indicate that on the label. Make sure any product you use actually contains sunscreen — many tanning oils and lotions don't.

Practice safe sex

We tend to associate sexually transmitted diseases with teenagers, but approximately half of these diseases are diagnosed in adults age 25 and older.

Sexually transmitted diseases (STDs) are on the increase in the United States. They include chlamydia infections, gonorrhea, genital herpes, venereal warts, syphilis and the human immunodeficiency virus (HIV), which causes AIDS.

Many of these diseases can be acquired during a single sexual encounter. Although HIV can also result from shared use of contaminated needles or, rarely, a blood transfusion, its main mode of transmission is sexual contact.

Most sexually transmitted diseases are treatable, but some have no cure and others can pose serious complications if not diagnosed early. To protect yourself:

Seek a monogamous relationship

The only sure ways of preventing a sexually transmitted disease are through sexual abstinence or a mutually monogamous relationship with an uninfected person. If you or your partner has or had several sexual partners — heterosexual or homosexual — or used intravenous drugs, you're at higher risk of contracting a disease.

Use condoms

Use of a condom during sexual intercourse doesn't eliminate the risk of acquiring or transmitting

a sexual disease, but it can significantly reduce the risk. The key is correct and consistent use. Condoms (prophylactics, or "rubbers") come in various thicknesses, colors and shapes. They may be lubricated or unlubricated, have a plain end or a reservoir end, and have a ribbed, smooth or corrugated texture.

When purchasing condoms, look for packages that mention protection of sexually transmitted diseases and check the expiration date. Condoms sometimes are made of animal membrane, but pores in this type of natural material may allow HIV to pass through. Latex condoms are recommended instead.

To be effective, a condom must be undamaged, applied to an erect penis before any genital contact and kept in place until it's removed on completion of sexual activity. Extra lubrication — even with lubricated condoms — can help prevent a condom from breaking. Use only water-based lubricants. Oil-based lubricants aren't recommended because they may cause a condom to break down.

After intercourse, the proper way to remove the condom is to hold on to it tightly at the rim and pull it off slowly while the penis is still hard, to prevent spillage of fluid.

A female condom also is available that can help reduce the risk of contracting a sexually transmitted disease. The availability of a female condom gives women more control over their personal health. Most forms of female-directed contraception, such as the pill or diaphragm, don't protect against disease transmission. However, studies indicate that use of a spermicide decreases the frequency of gonorrhea and chlamydial infections. Using a spermicide in conjunction with a diaphragm also may help kill bacteria.

Avoid certain sexual practices

Various sexual practices carry different degrees of risk of contracting a sexually transmitted disease.

Receptive (passive) anal intercourse is the riskiest behavior for acquiring HIV because it may damage the anal and rectal membranes and allows the virus to enter the bloodstream more easily. The passive partner is at much higher risk of contracting HIV than is the active partner, although an active partner can acquire gonorrhea and syphilis from infection in the passive partner's rectum.

Heterosexual vaginal intercourse, particularly with casual partners, also carries a risk of contracting HIV. The virus is believed to be more easily transmitted from the man to the woman than vice versa. This type of sexual activity is how most other sexually transmitted diseases are transmitted or acquired.

Oral sex isn't any safer. It also is a possible means of transmission of HIV, gonorrhea, herpes and other sexual diseases.

Activities that involve only skin-to-skin contact with no exposure to body fluids shouldn't spread disease.

Wear plugs and goggles

Life is generally more enjoyable when you can hear and see what's happening around you. Ear and eye injures often occur because proper safety precautions weren't taken.

Your ears

An estimated 28 million Americans have mild to severe hearing loss. As audio devices and systems become louder and more mobile, that number is likely to increase.

Exposure to loud noise over long periods — or even a single exposure to a very loud noise — can cause permanent hearing loss. To preserve your hearing:

Wear hearing protection

The best form of hearing protection is one that's worn correctly 100 percent of the time. Earplugs should fit snugly. Earmuff cushions should completely encircle the ear. Look for devices that meet federal safety standards.

Cotton balls aren't effective. They don't dampen noise well, and they could get stuck in your ears.

Turn it down

If someone is listening to music on a headset and you can identify the music being played, it's too loud. Don't turn up the stereo or TV to drown out other noise.

What a racket!

The loudness of a sound is measured in units called decibels. Repeated exposure to noise above 85 decibels can be dangerous. Hearing protection is required in workplace settings in which employees are exposed to noise that averages more than 90 decibels during an eight-hour day. But the workplace isn't the only setting for loud noise. Hazardous noise levels also occur with common recreational and household activities.

Noise source	Approximate decibels
Whisper	30
Normal conversation	60
Ringing telephone	80
Power lawn mower	90
Hair dryer	90
Bulldozer	105
Chain saw	110
Ambulance siren	120
Jet engine at takeoff	140
12-gauge shotgun blast	165

Source: National Institute for Occupational Safety and Health, Centers for Disease Control and Prevention, 2001

Take a break

If you can't get away from the noise, take frequent breaks. Intermittent exposure is less damaging than continuous exposure.

Your eyes

Myths about eye care are common. Warnings that reading in dim light or by flashlight or sitting too close to the television screen will damage your eyes aren't true. These activities may make your eyes feel tired, but they won't harm your vision.

Some of the most common injuries to the eyes are the result of accidents while doing everyday tasks. To protect your sight:

Wear safety goggles or glasses

Always wear eye protection when working with industrial chemicals, welding equipment and power tools. Also wear protective glasses or a face mask during certain sporting activities such as racquetball, squash, hockey and football, and when catcher in baseball and softball. Teach your children to do the same.

Watch out for dangerous toys

Keep young children away from toys that could lead to eye injury, such as BB guns or spring-loaded toys that shoot darts. Don't allow children to have fireworks.

Be careful around car batteries

Attaching jumper cables to a car battery can cause the battery to explode and release acid, which can get in your eyes.

Use chemicals wisely

Your home and garage are filled with potentially hazardous materials — everything from toilet cleaners to insecticides. In the workplace, there are regulations to help ensure safe use of chemicals. At home, there aren't.

Household chemicals

Common and potentially dangerous household products include:

- Cleaning products, especially those containing chloride bleach, ammonia and detergents
- Toilet and drain cleaners
- Products containing alcohol
- Bug sprays and plant insecticides

Make it a rule in your home that all hazardous items are kept on a high shelf or in a locked cabinet out of the reach of children.

When using household cleaners and insecticides, follow the directions on the label and don't use more of the product than recommended.

Also be careful not to spray the product — or cause it to splash — so that it gets into your eyes.

Workshop and yard chemicals

Common and potentially dangerous workshop and lawn and garden products include:

- Adhesives, glues, furniture strippers, stains and finishes
- Automotive products
- Herbicides, insecticides and fertilizers

Similar to indoor chemicals, store these products on a high shelf or in a locked cabinet.

When using such products, read the directions and take special precautions. Many chemicals are easily absorbed through the skin or harmful if you inhale them. You may want to wear rubber gloves and shoes, and long pants. Perhaps you should wear a breathing mask or respirator or protective goggles. If you're spraying a chemical, make sure the wind isn't blowing.

When finished with the product, dispose of it properly. This may involve bringing the item to the nearest hazardous waste disposal center. Don't put chemicals down the storm sewer, which goes into the city water supply.

Poison control center

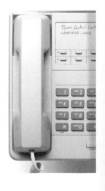

If you think someone has ingested a poison, or if you want to learn more about a potentially poisonous product, contact the American Association of Poison Control Centers. The toll-free number is (800) 222-1222. The Web site address is: *www.aapcc.org*.

Safeguard your home

Every year, tens of thousands of Americans die of injuries sustained in their own homes. A few simple steps can often prevent accidental injuries and deaths.

Store guns properly

If you keep a gun in your home, it should be stored without ammunition and locked in a secure cabinet that's out of the reach of children.

Maintain the weapon to prevent malfunction and acquaint yourself with the weapon's safety features and its unloading and loading procedures. More gun-related accidents occur in the home than anywhere else.

Check your smoke detectors

More than 2,000 people died in residential fires in 2002 (the latest figures available). In more than 60 percent of these fires, smoke alarms weren't present or weren't working.

Test your smoke detector monthly to make sure that the batteries are good, and change the batteries at least once a year. If your smoke detectors are wired to your home electrical system, make sure they have backup batteries.

Make sure you have a smoke detector on each level of your home. Locate smoke detectors on the ceiling in the sleeping areas of your home and in areas where fires are most likely to start, such as the kitchen or garage.

Place the smoke detector at least six inches from where the wall joins the ceiling. Avoid placing a detector in dead airspace, such as in a corner, where smoke may not reach it as quickly.

Purchase a fire extinguisher

Have a fire extinguisher in the kitchen. You might also keep additional ones in the garage and in the basement. Be sure members of your family know how to operate a fire extinguisher. Check the device annually.

Be aware of carbon monoxide

Carbon monoxide is tasteless, odorless, colorless and deadly. The risk of carbon monoxide poisoning is often greatest during cold weather, and is often due to defective control valves or pilot lights on cooking or heating units such as furnaces and portable kerosene space heaters.

Purchase a carbon monoxide detector for your home. It sounds a warning when carbon monoxide levels exceed safe levels. Look for the code UL 2034 on the box, indicating the detector meets industry standards.

To prevent carbon monoxide poisoning, make sure flame-burning appliances and fireplaces are properly installed and ventilated. And don't operate gas-powered motors in confined spaces, such as a closed garage or a basement.

Reduce the risk of falls

About half of falls happen at home. To make your home safer:

- Remove things you can trip over, such as papers and shoes, from stairs and places you walk.
- Avoid placing items in high locations that require use of a stool.
- When using ladders, make sure the ladder is in good condition and you have it properly positioned so it won't slip.

Reduce the risk of suffocation

Suffocation is a common cause of injury death among infants and children. To reduce risk of suffocation in the home.

- Make sure infants have a safe sleep environment. The mattress should be firm, and don't place comforters, thick blankets, pillows or stuffed toys in the sleep area.
- Make sure toy chests have ventilation holes that can't become blocked and don't let children play near unused appliances.
- Warn children about the dangers of automobile trunks.

Index